Practical Coronary Thrombolysis

David de Bono
MA, MD, FRCP(Ed)
British Heart Foundation,
Professor of Cardiology,
University of Leicester,
Leicester, UK

Blackwell Scientific Publications
OXFORD LONDON EDINBURGH
BOSTON MELBOURNE

Editorial Offices:
Osney Mead, Oxford OX2 0EL
25 John Street, London WC1N 2BL
23 Ainslie Place, Edinburgh EH3 6AJ
3 Cambridge Center, Suite 208
Cambridge, Massachusetts 02142
USA
107 Barry Street, Carlton
Victoria 3053, Australia

First published 1990

Set by Setrite Typesetters, Hong Kong
Printed and bound in Great Britain
by Billing & Sons Ltd, Worcester

DISTRIBUTORS

Marston Book Services Ltd
PO Box 87
Oxford OX2 0DT
(*Orders*: Tel: 0865 791155
Fax: 0865 791927
Telex: 837515)

USA
Year Book Medical Publishers
200 North LaSalle Street
Chicago, Illinois 60601
(*Orders*: Tel: (312) 726-9733)

Canada
The C.V. Mosby Company
5240 Finch Avenue East
Scarborough, Ontario
(*Orders*: Tel: (416) 298-1588)

Australia
Blackwell Scientific Publications
(Australia) Pty Ltd
107 Barry Street
Carlton, Victoria 3053
(*Orders*: Tel: (03) 347-0300)

British Library
Cataloguing in Publication Data

de Bono, David
Practical coronary thrombolysis.
1. Man. Heart. Muscles.
Infarction. Drug therapy
I. title
616.1'237061

ISBN 0-632-02705-3

Contents

Introduction

The pathology of coronary thrombosis has been recognized for over a century; the thrombolytic effect of streptococcal culture filtrates was described in 1934 and streptokinase first used clinically in 1947; and the first trial of thrombolysis in myocardial infarction was attempted in 1958. Yet it is only in the last decade that the efficacy of thrombolytic therapy in patients with coronary thrombosis has been established beyond doubt, and its central role in treating these patients acknowledged. The sheer speed of advance of knowledge, the plethora of publications, the involvement of much 'high-tech' cardiology and the understandable enthusiasm of different pharmaceutical companies for their own thrombolytic agents have been exhilarating but also confusing. This book is intended to be a simple and practical guide to thrombolytic therapy in acute myocardial infarction. It is written for, and dedicated to, the doctors and nurses who actually treat myocardial infarct patients, whether in the accident and emergency department, in the CCU, or on general medical wards. It is meant both for background reading and for reference.

The first three chapters give the historical background to the development of thrombolytic therapy, explain how the different thrombolytic drugs work, and discuss the clinical trial data on the efficacy of coronary thrombolysis.

The following chapters (4–16) discuss in practical terms the selection of patients, the administration of thrombolytic and adjustment therapy, the assessment and follow-up of patients after thrombolysis, and the immediate and longer-term problems which may arise. The use of thrombolytic therapy for other medical problems is also discussed.

The Appendix contains a selection of flow-charts and check-lists for rapid reference.

I have indicated some sources of further reading at the end of each chapter: in general these are either authoritative and well-referenced reviews, or the definitive reports of the original trials on which our knowledge of clinical thrombolysis is based.

DdeB
June 1989

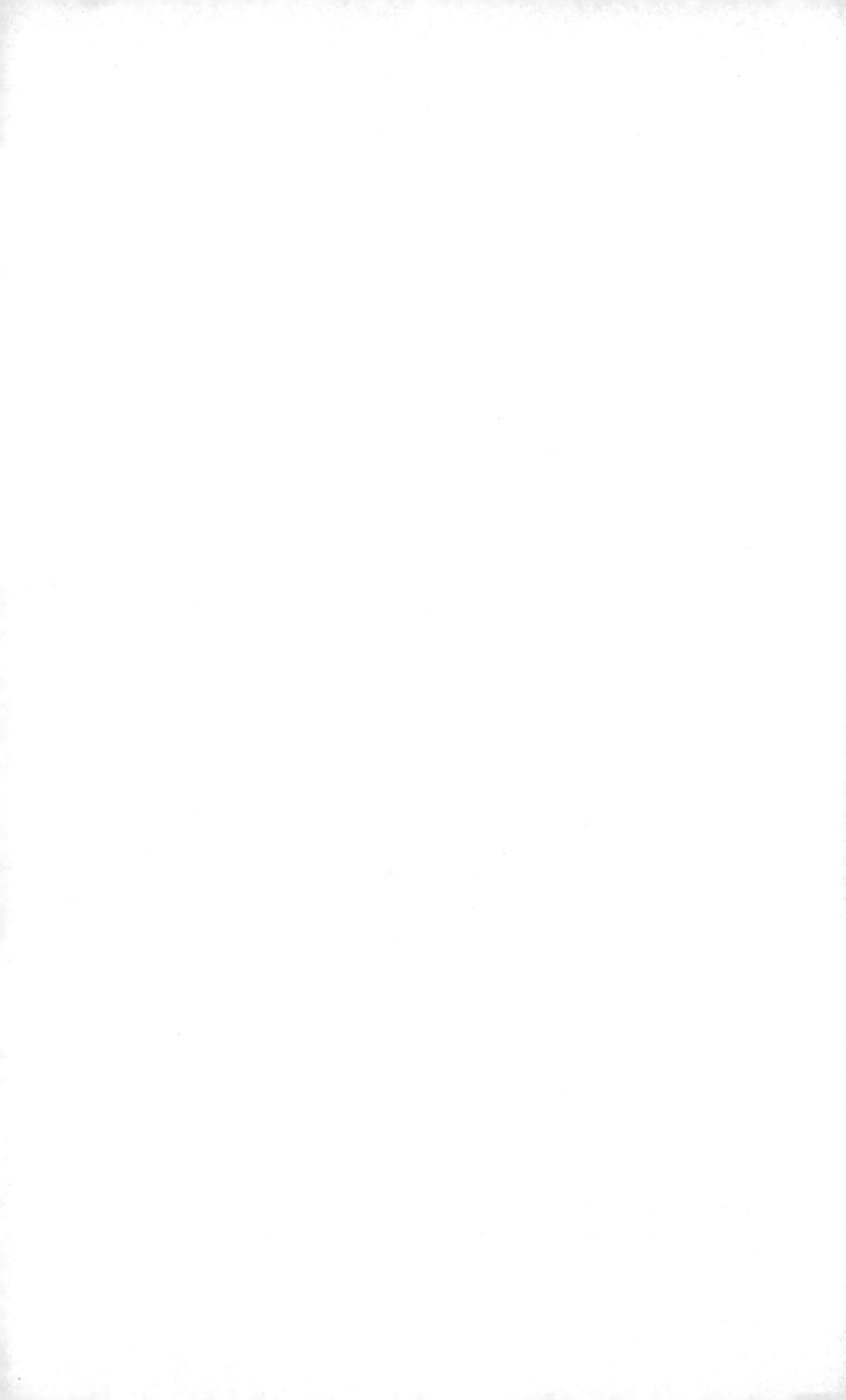

1: The Cause of Myocardial Infarction

Myocardial infarction is usually due to the thrombotic occlusion of a coronary artery. The thrombus nearly always starts at the site of a cracked or disrupted atheromatous plaque (Fig. 1.1). Small cracks in a plaque lead to haemorrhage into the intima, but the crack often seals over without further problems. In more extensive cracks, platelet activation takes place, leading to narrowing of the vessel lumen and possibly to an element of arterial spasm. An unstable flap of intima may lead to further obstruction.

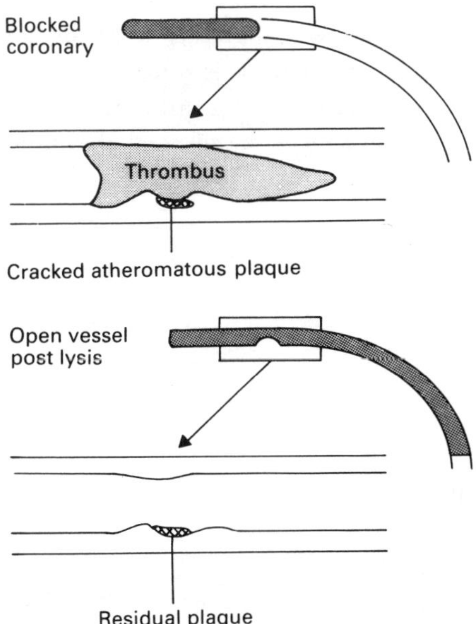

Fig. 1.1 Diagram to show the relationship between a cracked atheromatous plaque and occlusive coronary thrombus.

The precise mechanism which first leads to the formation of an intraluminal, occlusive fibrin thrombus is still uncertain, but once formed, intraluminal thrombus may propagate rapidly. Retrograde propagation usually extends to the first major side branch before the block, antegrade propagation is more variable, though it may be extensive (Fig. 1.2). In a proportion of patients, occlusion may be intermittent, perhaps as thrombus builds up and breaks away. Some of them go on to develop total occlusion, while in others the process somehow stabilizes and the vessel remains patent.

The immediate consequence of coronary occlusion is myocardial ischaemia, leading to anginal pain, impaired contractility, arrhythmias and eventually myocardial cell death. In dogs, sudden total occlusion of a major coronary artery leads to progressive infarction, such that restoration of flow after 3 hours or longer is unable to restore any significant function. In other species, the existence of a collateral circulation may preserve myocardium for longer periods. In man, occlusion of a chronically-stenosed vessel with well-established collaterals to the distal vessel seldom causes infarction. However there is some evidence that vasoconstrictor substances released from a thrombus may actually delay or inhibit the development of a collateral circulation after acute coronary thrombosis.

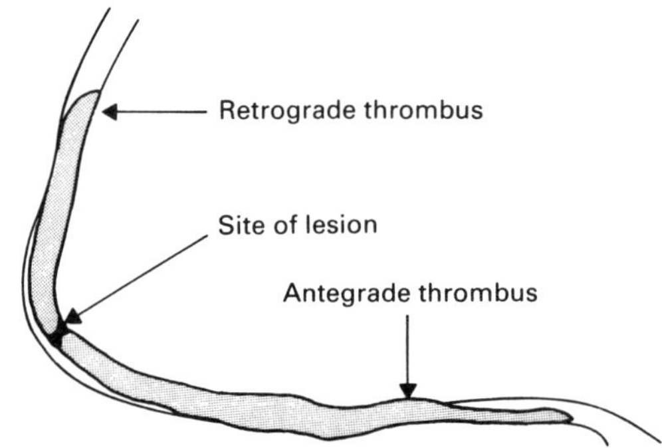

Fig. 1.2 Diagram to show retrograde and antegrade propagation of thrombus from the initial lesion.

Why does myocardium die as a result of ischaemia? The traditional, and simplest view is that because myocardial cells are committed to aerobic respiration, their continued efforts to contract under ischaemic conditions lead to a progressive and ultimately fatal depletion of energy substrates such as ATP. This is almost certainly an over-simplification. One of the earliest effects of ischaemia is a depression of myocardial contractility, and coincidentally of energy consumption, and this should help protect the myocardium. Moreover, in some situations where coronary flow is cut off and then restored after a period of ischaemia, the morphological features of cell damage either do not appear until, or at least develop much more rapidly after, reperfusion. The concept of reperfusion injury is controversial: some authorities maintain that it is an important mechanism for myocardial damage, and that much of the injury is done by free radicals produced as a result of a sudden rise in oxygen tension in tissues whose normal protection against these substances has been depressed. Others contend that the damage was done during ischaemia, and we are simply seeing its delayed effects after reperfusion. This is not simply an academic point, for if we knew how ischaemia caused damage we would be in a better position to protect against it.

A further area of uncertainty is whether the damage caused by ischaemia is done at the level of the heart muscle cells, or at the level of the endothelium of the cardiac capillaries. After fairly prolonged periods of ischaemia, even the removal of the block in the coronary artery causes poor flow downstream; the 'no reflow' phenomenon. There is evidence that a major component of the no reflow phenomenon is due to excessive plugging of cardiac capillaries with polymorphonuclear leukocytes, and if these are excluded, the phenomenon is suppressed and myocardial salvage is improved. Recent experiments suggest that different mechanisms may damage the cardiac muscle cells (predominantly ischaemia) and the vascular endothelial cells (predominantly reperfusion injury).

Although the concepts of reperfusion injury and of protection against ischaemic damage are interesting and challenging, there is at present little evidence for their relevance to the clinical situation. All the clinical trials of thrombolytic therapy in human myocardial infarction have emphasized that the earlier reperfusion is achieved, the better the likely outcome, both in terms of survival and of improved left ventricular function.

Unstable angina

This is a clinical condition in which episodes of myocardial ischaemia occur at rest or on minimal exertion. In many patients it is due to rupture of an atheromatous plaque with thrombus formation which narrows, but does not completely occlude the lumen. Unstable angina can be regarded either as myocardial infarction occurring over an unusually extended timescale, or as the consequence of plaque rupture under conditions relatively unfavorable to the formation of occlusive thrombus. In either case, timely intervention may help preserve coronary patency and prevent progression to infarction.

Subendocardial infarction

This is an electrocardiographic diagnosis based on the ECG findings of T wave inversion and no Q wave development as opposed to the ST segment elevation and Q waves of 'transmural' infarction. The most common angiographic finding is of a patent but severely stenosed coronary vessel, and it is likely that many cases of subendocardial infarction are due to transient occlusion and early reperfusion.

Non-thrombotic causes of myocardial infarction are rare. They include coronary spasm, either spontaneous or drug-induced, embolism from fragments of endocarditic vegetation or intracardiac thrombus, and sudden severe rises in blood pressure as in phaeochromocytoma. The history and physical examination usually give some clues to the diagnosis.

Summary

- Most infarcts are due to thrombotic occlusion of a coronary artery.

- Thrombus formation is usually associated with a cracked atheromatous plaque.
- The plaque which leads to thrombus formation need not have caused severe obstruction previously.
- Factors which lead to the initial cracking or rupture of the atheromatous plaque are poorly understood, but may include vigorous physical exertion.
- Obstruction is often intermittent, at least in the early stages.
- The longer the occlusion, the more severe the myocardial damage.
- The roles of reperfusion injury and of free radicals in ischaemic damage are presently under investigation.
- Unstable angina is often associated with plaque cracking and thrombus formation, but occlusive thrombus is rare.
- Subendocardial infarction may be the result of a brief period of coronary occlusion.

Further reading

Ambrose, J.A., Winters, S.L. & Stern, A. (1986) Angiographic evolution of coronary artery morphology in unstable angina. *Journal of the American College of Cardiology*, **7**, 472–478.

Bernier, M., Hearse, D.J. & Manning, A.S. (1986) Reperfusion induced arrhythmias and oxygen-induced free radicals: studies with anti-free radical interventions and a free radical generating system in the isolated perfused rat heart. *Circulation Research*, **58**, 331–340.

Davies, M.J. & Thomas, A.C. (1985) Plaque fissuring: the cause of acute myocardial infarction, sudden ischaemic death and crescendo angina. *British Heart Journal*, **53**, 363–373.

Davies, M.J., Woolf, N. & Robertson, W.B. (1976) Pathology of acute myocardial infarction with particular reference to occlusive coronary thrombi. *British Heart Journal*, **38**, 659–664.

DeWood, M.A., Spores, J., Notske, R. *et al.* (1980) Prevalence of total coronary occlusion during the early hours of transmural myocardial infarction. *New England Journal of Medicine*, **303**, 897–902.

DeWood, M.A., Stifter, W.F., Simpson, C.S. *et al.* (1986) Coronary arteriographic findings soon after non-Q-wave myocardial infarction. *New England Journal of Medicine*, **315**, 417–423.

Sherman, C.T., Litvack, F., Grundfest, W. *et al.* (1986) Coronary angioscopy in patients with unstable angina. *New England Journal of Medicine,* **315**, 913–919.

2: How Thrombolysis Works

In order to understand thrombolysis, we need to understand the structure of a thrombus (Fig. 2.1). A thrombus is defined as the product of blood coagulation in a flowing blood stream (as distinct from a clot, which can form under conditions of stasis, or after death). Thrombi usually contain fibrin, platelets, leukocytes, red cells and a number of other plasma-derived proteins. Fibrin is an insoluble protein which can be regarded as a kind of cement or glue, holding the thrombus together. Soluble plasma

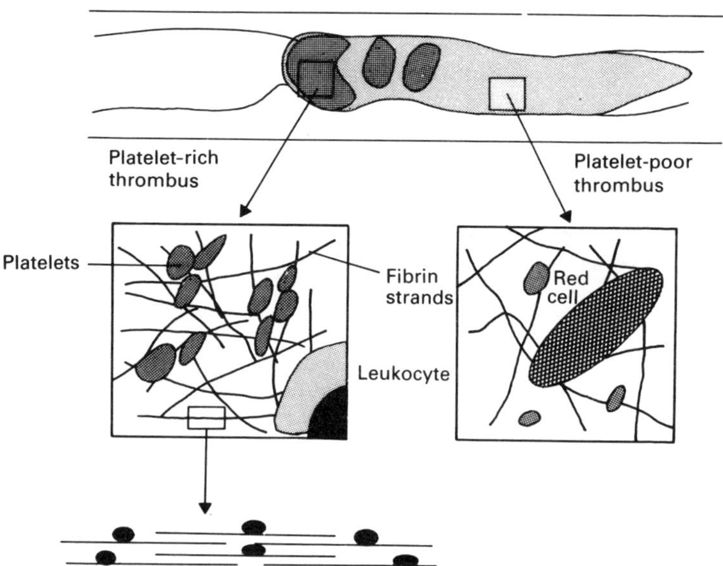

Fig. 2.1 Diagram of the structure of a thrombus.

fibrinogen is converted to fibrin by the action of the proteolytic enzyme thrombin, which specifically cleaves a single bond in the fibrinogen molecule. The fibrin molecules then line up to form insoluble strands of fibrin. In a short while, these strands are stabilized by cross-link formation between lysine residues in the fibrin chain. Although cell to cell adhesion among platelets or leukocytes may play a role in the formation of the thrombus, its stability over periods of hours or days is almost entirely dependent on fibrin. Eventually, unless the thrombus is dissolved, it becomes 'organized' by the ingrowth of fibroblasts and smooth muscle cells, which lay down collagen and other 'structural' proteins (Fig. 2.2).

In theory, fibrin might be broken up by any of a series of proteolytic enzymes. In practice, non-specific proteolytic enzymes are too toxic to use therapeutically, and if used in low doses would be inactivated by the protease inhibitors normally present in plasma. The body produces its own highly effective and specific fibrin-digesting protease (plasmin), which normally circulates in the plasma as an inactive precursor (plasminogen). Plasminogen binds strongly to fibrin, using specialized parts of its molecular structure called 'kringles' (Fig. 2.3). Under normal circumstances every fibrin thrombus that forms in the body

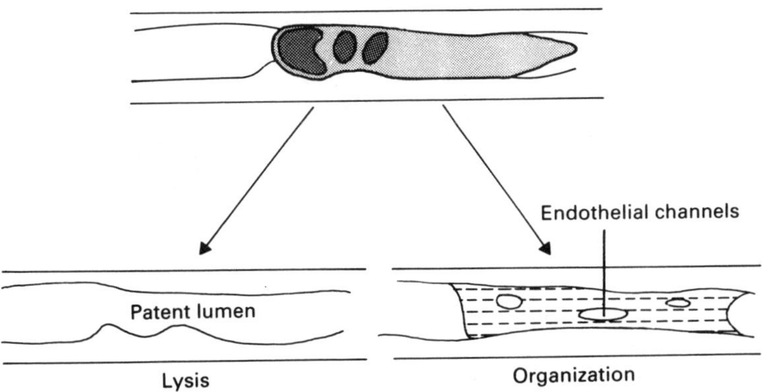

Fig. 2.2 Diagram to show the organization of thrombus by ingrowing fibroblasts and smooth muscle levels.

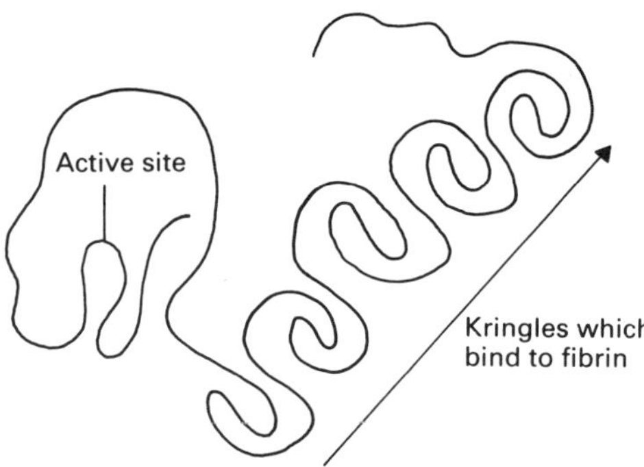

Fig. 2.3 Diagram of the molecular structure of plasminogen.

incorporates plasminogen, in an approximately 1 : 1 molecular ratio with fibrin. All the currently available thrombolytic drugs work not by digesting fibrin directly, but by activating plasminogen to plasmin (Fig. 2.4).

Plasmin digests fibrin into a series of smaller molecules (fibrin degradation products or FDPs) which are cleared by the reticulo-endothelial system or, in some cases, excreted in the urine. Although plasmin*ogen* has a higher affinity for fibrin than for

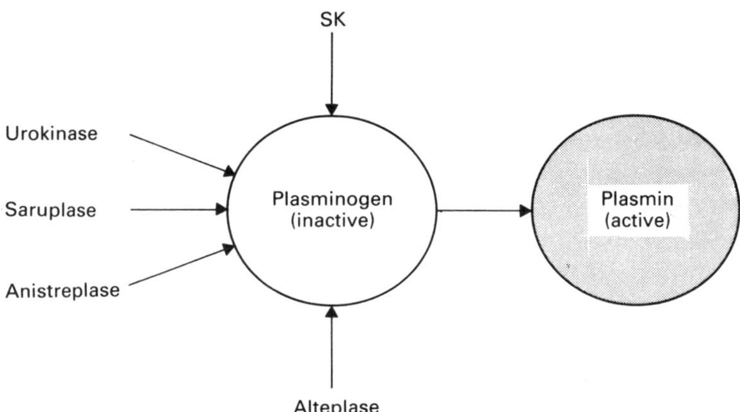

Fig. 2.4 All currently available thrombolytic drugs act by causing the activation of plasminogen to plasmin.

fibrinogen, it is possible for circulating plasminogen to become activated, and the resulting circulating plasmin may degrade free circulating fibrinogen as well as thrombus-bound fibrin. The body can cope with small amounts of free plasmin in the circulation by mopping it up with α_2-antiplasmin, but large quantities of free plasmin will overwhelm this mechanism, and lead to a marked depletion of plasma fibrinogen (Fig. 2.5). This may lead to excessive bleeding, partly because of the lack of fibrinogen and partly because some of the fibrin degradation products actually have some heparin-like anticoagulant activity.

Streptokinase

Streptokinase was the first thrombolytic drug to be studied. It was identified in filtrates from cultures of *Streptococcus pyogenes*, and it is not a natural body product. Streptokinase activates circulating or fibrin-bound plasminogen indiscriminately. The streptokinase molecule forms a complex with the plasminogen which alters the conformation of the plasminogen, and thus leads to it becoming enzymatically active. The active complex can then activate other plasminogen molecules by proteolytic cleavage, setting off a chain reaction of activation (Fig. 2.6). It is characteristic of streptokinase (and urokinase, see below) that they cause both thrombolysis by activating fibrin-bound plasminogen and systemic fibrinogenolysis by activating free circulating plasminogen.

Anistreplase

Another effect of the change in shape of the plasminogen molecule when it forms a complex with streptokinase is that it develops a much increased affinity for fibrin. This was taken advantage of in the design of the 'second generation' thrombolytic drug anistreplase (Fig. 2.7). Here, a mixture of streptokinase and human plasminogen is allowed to react and form complexes outside the body, in the hope that these will form a 'fibrin-selective' thrombolytic agent. As mentioned above, the formation of the complex will activate the enzymic site of plasminogen, and it is necessary to 'block' this as otherwise activation of circulating plasminogen

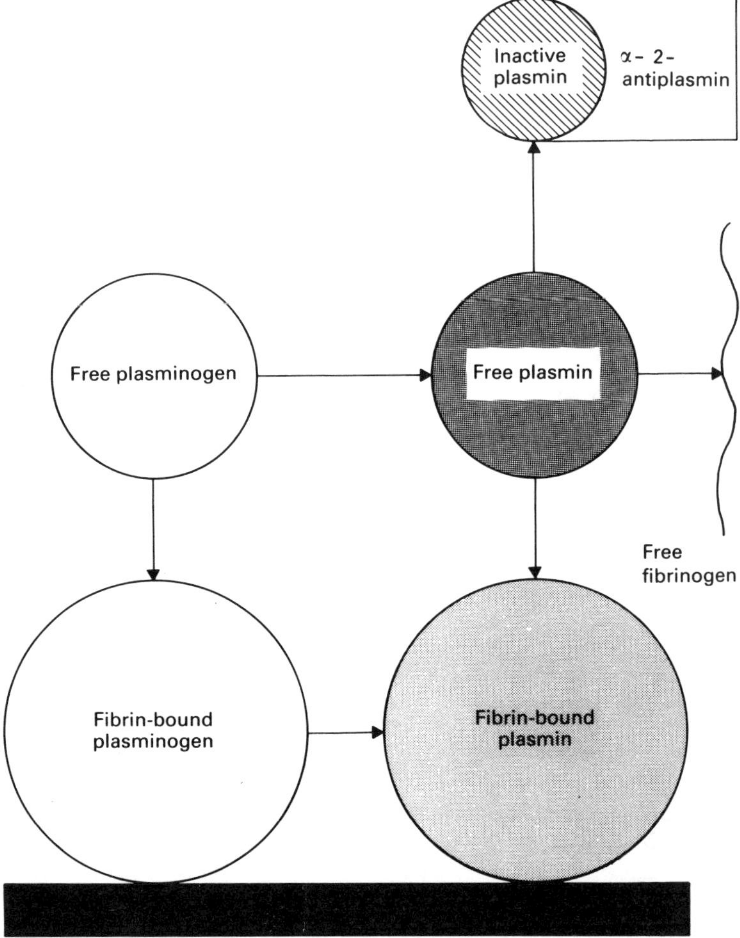

Fig. 2.5 Some thrombolytic drugs preferentially activate fibrin-bound plasminogen (alteplase, saruplase, anistreplase), whilst others (streptokinase, urokinase) activate free and bound plasminogen indiscriminately. Free circulating plasmin can be inactivated by α-2-antiplasmin, but there is not enough of this to inactivate all the circulating plasmin produced by a 'non-selective' fibrinolytic agent.

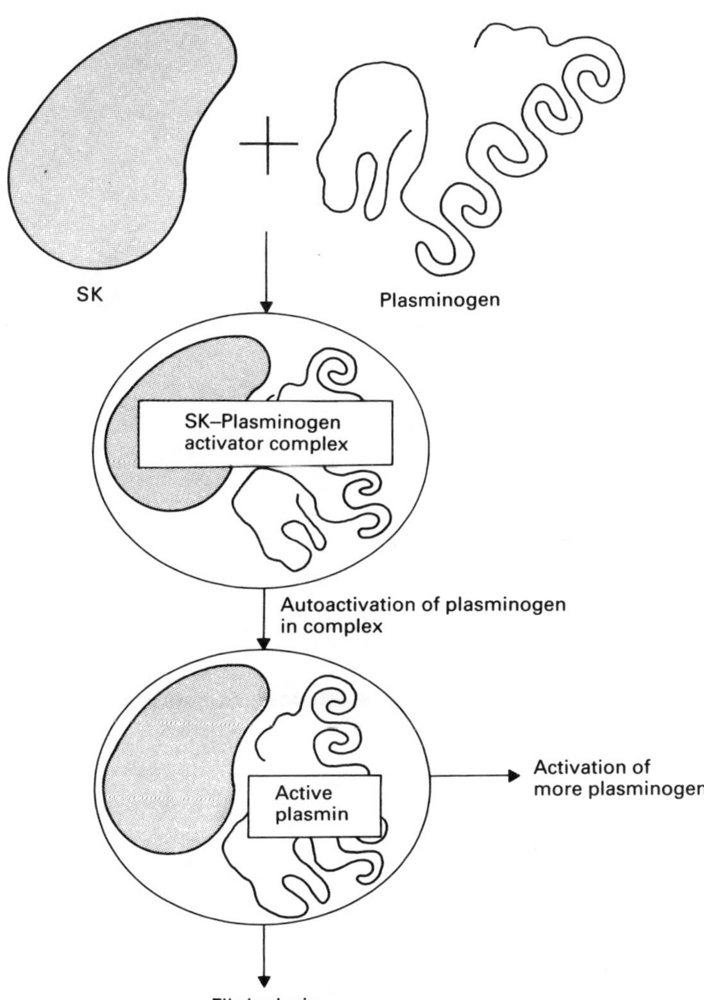

Fig. 2.6 Streptokinase activates plasminogen by binding to it and forming an 'activator complex'. The conformational change induced by the streptokinase causes the plasminogen to become enzymically active, and the complex can activate further plasminogen molecules by cleaving a peptide bond.

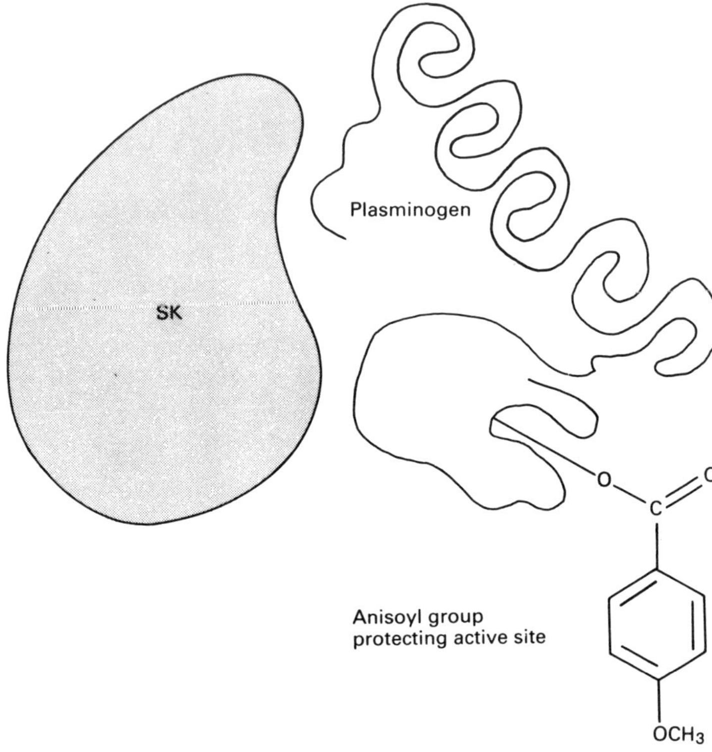

Fig. 2.7 Diagram of the structure of anistreplase (anisoylated plasminogen–streptokinase activator complex).

will take place as soon as the complex is injected. The blocking is accomplished by esterifying the active site to an anisoyl group—this hydrolyses away with a half-life of about 36 minutes in aqueous solution at body temperature. An unexpected but welcome consequence of complexing streptokinase with 'blocked' plasminogen is that the complex is less likely to activate other enzyme systems such as the kallikrein/kallidin system, and can thus be injected rapidly without causing hypotension.

Tissue plasminogen activator (alteplase)

Tissue type plasminogen activator (t-PA, known pharmaceutically as alteplase) differs fundamentally from streptokinase and urokinase in its structure (Fig. 2.8). It is a naturally occurring mammalian protein, made in minute quantities in many tissues, but particularly in the vascular endothelium. In many tissues it is produced in parallel with an inhibitor (plasminogen activator inhibitor, PAI) which inactivates it by forming a complex. The factors controlling the physiological balance between fibrinolytic activation and inhibition are incompletely understood. There is pronounced diurnal variation in fibrinolytic activity, with a marked trough in the early morning, and fibrinolytic activity is stimulated by vascular distension (e.g. blowing up a sphygmomanometer cuff) or physical exercise, sometimes with a rebound depression of activity afterwards. t-PA is a proteolytic enzyme which activates plasminogen by cleaving a specific peptide bond.

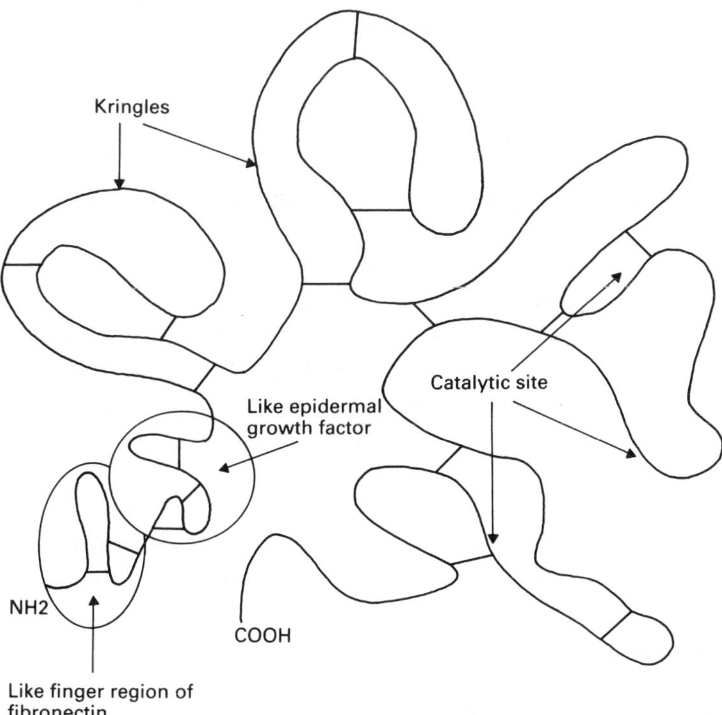

Fig. 2.8 Secondary structure of altepase (tissue-type plasminogen activator).

It has a low affinity for circulating plasminogen, but binds much more effectively to plasminogen in the presence of fibrin—it is thus, at least to some extent, a 'fibrin-specific' thrombolytic.

In biochemical terms, the affinity of an enzyme for its substrate is measured by the Michaelis constant *K*m, which is the concentration of substrate necessary for a given quantity of enzyme to work at half its maximum rate. With t-PA, the *K*m for free plasminogen is nearly 100 times the *K*m for plasminogen in the presence of fibrin. Remember however that 'pharmacological' concentrations of drugs may be several orders of magnitude greater than the physiological concentrations of the same agents.

Urokinase

Urokinase is a naturally occurring plasminogen activator first identified in urine. It is a proteolytic enzyme which activates plasminogen by a specific cleavage of a single peptide bond. Despite its different mode of action its clinical effect is very similar to that of streptokinase, with indiscriminate activation of both circulating and fibrin-bound plasminogen.

Saruplase (single chain urokinase type plasminogen activator, SCU-PA)

This agent is presently available only for experimental use. It is a naturally occurring thrombolytic agent which has considerable structural homology with urokinase, but SCU-PA is a larger molecule, molecular weight 55 000. Following limited proteolytic cleavage, it develops urokinase-like proteolytic and plasminogen activating abilities. In the presence of plasma and a fibrin clot, thrombolytic activity develops after a short lag phase, but saruplase is not spontaneously active in plasma alone. Limited clinical trials indicate it is an effective thrombolytic agent in terms of coronary patency, but systemic fibrinogen degradation does occur.

Summary

- Thrombi are held together by fibrin.
- As thrombi age, increasing amounts of fibrin cross-linking occur.

- Plasmin is the principal enzyme for digesting fibrin.
- Plasminogen, the inactive precursor of plasmin, circulates in the plasma and becomes incorporated into thrombi.
- All currently available thrombolytic drugs work by activating plasminogen. Urokinase and streptokinase activate free and fibrin-bound plasminogen indiscriminately, anistreplase and alteplase preferentially activate fibrin-bound plasminogen.

Further reading

Collen, D., Stump, D.C. & Gold, H.K. (1988) Thrombolytic therapy. *Annual Review of Medicine*, **39**, 405–423.

Marder, V.J. & Sherry, S. (1988) Thrombolytic therapy: current status. *New England Journal of Medicine*, **318**, 1512–1520, 1585–1595.

3: Clinical Trials of Thrombolysis in Myocardial Infarction

The object of this chapter is not to give an exhaustive account of every clinical trial involving thrombolysis in infarction, but to explain as concisely as possible the scientific basis for our present use of coronary thrombolysis. It is important to remember that a good clinical trial is designed to provide a convincing answer to a defined question or group of questions: trying to extrapolate beyond these limits by data dredging or other means is likely to be misleading.

Evidence that thrombolytic therapy improves survival

The first reported clinical trial of intravenous streptokinase in myocardial infarction was reported by Fletcher, Alkjaersig, Smyrniotis and Sherry in 1959. It demonstrated that such therapy was practicable, but was too small to demonstrate any convincing benefit. A large number of intravenous streptokinase trials were performed over the succeeding two decades; in retrospect they also were too small to produce convincing endpoints, but an overview or 'meta-analysis' by Yusuf and colleagues in 1985 detected an overall mortality reduction of about 20% in patients randomized to thrombolytic therapy. This meta-analysis had a major impact on the subsequent International Study of Infarct Survival (ISIS)-2 study. One of the trials, by Breddin and colleagues in 1973, was significant in that it introduced the concept of 'high dose, short duration' treatment with streptokinase. Perhaps the most convincing of this 'early' phase of trials was the European Cooperative Study Group (ECSG) trial published in 1979 whose results are summarized in Fig. 3.1.

This study showed that in a preselected 'high-risk' group of patients, thrombolytic therapy reduced 30-day mortality from

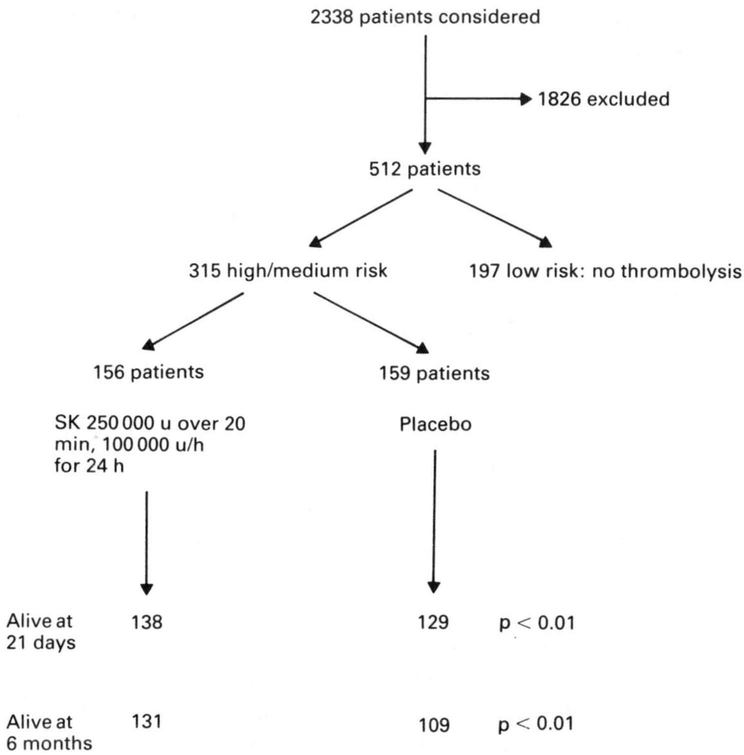

Fig. 3.1 European cooperative trial of streptokinase in myocardial infarction: 1979. (From Verstraete, M., van de Loo, J. & Jesdinsky, H.J. (1981) *Acta Medica Scandinavica*, Supplement **648**, 1–56.)

30% in the control group to 16% in the treated group. It was criticised (unfairly) for the relatively small proportion of patients registered who were actually admitted to the study, and (fairly) for the high proportions of major bleeding complications resulting from a prolonged (24-hour) thrombolytic regime.

The logical descendants of this trial are the Gruppo Italiano per lo Studio della Streptochinasi nell' Infarto miocardico (GISSI) and ISIS-2 studies to be described below, but a digression is necessary here to consider the impact of intracoronary thrombolytic therapy and of the angiographic assessment of thrombolysis. Intracoronary thrombolysis had been considered in 1960, but the technical problems of selective intracoronary injection had not then been overcome. When Sones introduced coronary angiography in 1962 he was understandably anxious it should not get a bad reputation from indiscriminate use in high-risk patients, and angiography in patients with acute infarction was actively discouraged. Ruda and Chazov in the Soviet Union reinvented the concept of intracoronary administration of thrombolytic drugs in the mid-1970s, but their work was not widely known in the West until it was taken up by Rentrop in Berlin. In a parallel development, DeWood and colleagues in the USA were undertaking coronary arteriography in acute infarction with a view to referral for surgical revascularization. Their paper published in 1980 had two major effects: it settled the argument about whether coronary thrombosis caused myocardial infarction (see Chapter 1) and it made the Western cardiological world realize that coronary angiography in acute infarction was not unduly hazardous.

For the first time, coronary angiography provided a thrombolytic endpoint, the opening of a previously occluded artery, which was both unequivocal and could be measured in every patient studied. This was particularly important because newer thrombolytic agents were being developed (see Chapter 2) and needed to be tested. Supplies of such agents were far too limited for large scale studies with a mortality endpoint. At the same time, it was hoped that intracoronary administration of a small dose of streptokinase would reduce the bleeding complications associated with prolonged streptokinase therapy.

The Western Washington study (Fig. 3.2) was the first (and only) study of *intracoronary* streptokinase to show a significant mortality reduction in treated patients as compared with controls. Even as it was being conducted, Schröder was showing that an intravenous infusion of streptokinase 1 500 000 units over 60 minutes was also capable of producing a high rate of angiographic coronary patency, with the added advantage that such treatment could be initiated in the emergency room without waiting for a catheter laboratory to become available. Recognition of the compelling arguments for reperfusion as early as possible led to a mid-trial modification of the protocol for the Netherlands

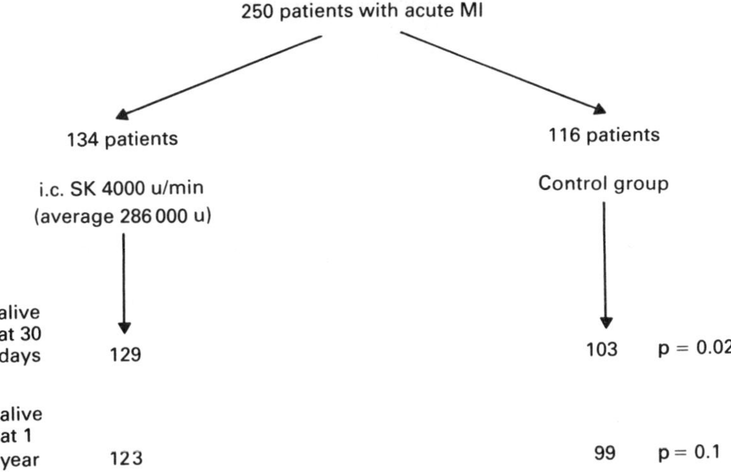

Fig. 3.2 The Western Washington trial of intracoronary streptokinase in acute myocardial infarction. (From Ward Kennedy, J., Ritchie, J.L., Davis, K.B. *et al.* (1985) *New England Journal of Medicine*, **312**, 1073–1078.)

Inter-University Institute trial (Fig. 3.3) from intracoronary streptokinase to intravenous streptokinase followed by coronary angiography and if necessary, mechanical recanalization plus angioplasty. This trial did not show a statistically different difference in survival between thrombolysis and control groups, but did show differences in the 'surrogate endpoints' of infarct size and left ventricular function. Arguments as to whether such surrogate endpoints could validly be used to predict mortality were, temporarily, interrupted by the publication of the GISSI trial.

THE GISSI STUDY

This was a large, simply designed study in which patients with clinical and ECG features of infarction were randomized to receive either conventional (non-thrombolytic) therapy or intravenous streptokinase 1 500 000 units over 1 hour (Fig. 3.4). The principal endpoints were mortality at 21 days and at 1 year after admission. 5852 patients were randomized to no thrombolytic treatment and the 21-day mortality was 13.0%, and 5860 to

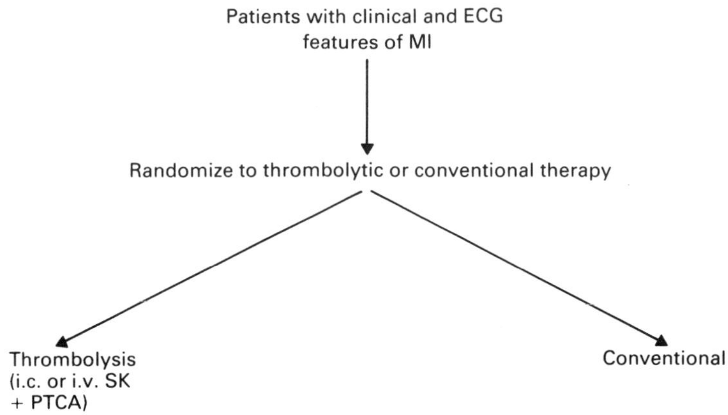

	Infarct size (median HBD release)	LV ejection fraction (%)
Conventional	1100 u/l	53
Thrombolysis	770 u/l	47

Fig. 3.3 Netherlands Inter-University Institute trial. (From Serruys, P.W. *et al.* (1986) *Journal of the American College of Cardiology*, **7**, 729–747, and Simoons, M.L. *et al.* ibid, 717–728.)

streptokinase, with a 21-day mortality of 10.7%. Overall, the relative mortality reduction was 18% with 95% confidence intervals of 10–28%. Prospective stratification of patients into those presenting at different times showed that the mortality reduction was most striking in those who presented early, with marginal evidence of benefit for those presenting after 6 hours and no benefit (indeed a worse outcome) after 12 hours (Table 3.1). In a trial of this size it is possible to assess fairly accurately the incidence of side-effects. Of patients given streptokinase, 3.7% had bleeding complications, and 1.1% had strokes.

THE ISIS-2 STUDY

This was a large trial which compared in double blind fashion the effect on survival of streptokinase (1 500 000 units over 1 hour), aspirin (160 mg daily), both or neither (Fig. 3.5).

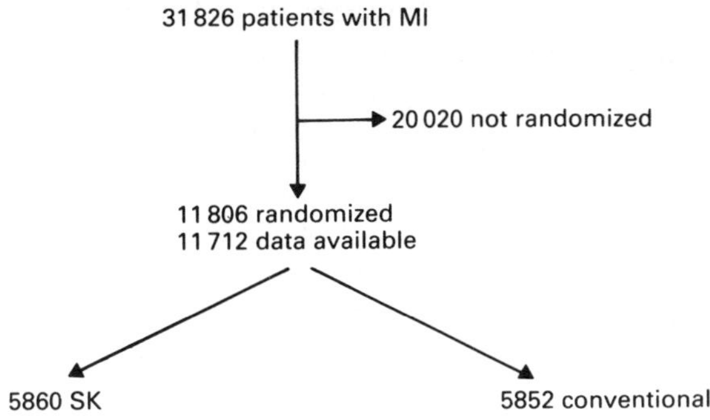

21-day mortality 628 (10.7%) 758 (13.0%)

Fig. 3.4 The GISSI trial of thrombolysis. (From GISSI study group (1986) *Lancet*, **i**, 397–401.)

Table 3.1 Effects of delay between onset of symptoms and treatment on survival in the GISSI-1 study.

	Mortality (within 1 month)		
Delay in treatment*	Streptokinase group	Control group	
<1 hour	8.2%	15.4%	p = <0.0001
<3 hours	9.2%	12.0%	p = <0.0005
>3–6 hours	11.7%	14.1%	p = <0.03
>6–9 hours	12.6%	14.1%	NS
>9–12 hours	15.8%	13.6%	NS

* Retrospective stratification.
Data from GISSI (1986) *Lancet*, **i**, 397.

Unlike GISSI, ECG criteria were not required for entry. The overall mortality in the 'double placebo' group at 5 weeks was 13%, and in the streptokinase alone group 10.3% — very similar to GISSI. Interestingly, aspirin had an independent effect on mortality (5-week mortality 10.7%), and the results with streptokinase and aspirin together were better than with either alone (5-week mortality 7.9%). The overall percentage reduction in mortality comparing streptokinase plus aspirin against double placebo was 41% (95% confidence intervals 33%–49%).

The combination of evidence from the early European studies, from the overview of smaller trials, and from GISSI and ISIS-2 makes an overwhelming case for the efficacy of thrombolytic therapy in reducing mortality in acute myocardial infarction. This is further emphasized by the evidence that the mortality reduction is not transient, but is sustained at 1 year.

Evidence for the relative benefit of different regimes

Having established that thrombolytic therapy with intravenous streptokinase is effective in improving survival, the most logical and convincing way to show that a new thrombolytic agent was superior would be to compare the two in a prospective, randomized trial large enough to use survival as an endpoint. This approach has a number of snags. We know that such a trial will have to be very large indeed, because the difference between two

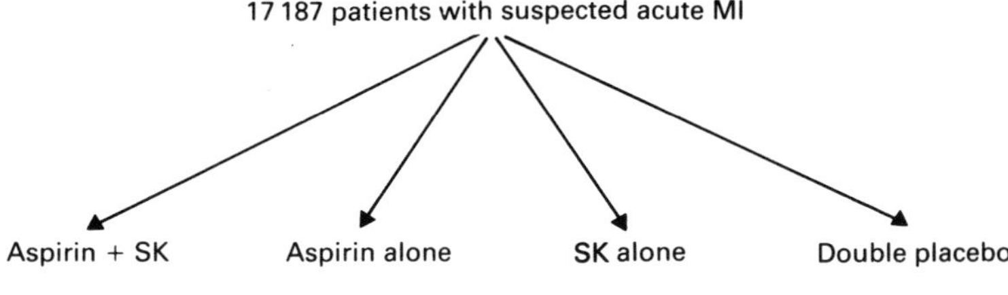

5-week vascular mortality:

	Number	Deaths (%)
All allocated to SK	8592	791 (9.2)
All allocated to SK placebo	8595	1029 (12.0)
All allocated to aspirin	8587	804 (9.4)
All allocated to aspirin placebo	8600	1016 (11.8)
All allocated to SK + aspirin	4292	343 (8.0)
Allocated to double placebo	4300	568 (13.2)

Fig. 3.5 Second international study of infarct survival (ISIS-2). (From ISIS-2 Collaborative Group (1988) *Lancet*, **ii**, 349–360.)

effective agents will be much less than between a single agent and placebo, and because the 'control group' mortality is likely to be low. It would be difficult or impossible to use such a trial to compare different doses, so it would be important to make the right choice of dose schedule for the new drug. The trial would inevitably be very expensive. For all these reasons, preliminary trials of new thrombolytic drugs have invariably used 'surrogate endpoints' such as coronary patency or left ventricular function. Examples are the Thrombolysis in Myocardial Infarction (TIMI)-1 study and the ECSG-2 study comparing streptokinase and alteplase, the German Activator Urokinase (GAU) study comparing alteplase and urokinase, and the Pro-Urokinase in Myocardial Infarction (PRIMI) study comparing streptokinase and SCU-PA. All these are discussed in Chapter 6. This type of study can also be used for dose ranging.

In general, regulatory authorities such as the Committee for Safety of Medicines in the UK and the Food and Drug Administration in the USA have been sceptical about accepting surrogate endpoints as 'proof of efficacy' of new agents. Manufacturers have therefore felt compelled to mount placebo-controlled trials of new drugs to provide evidence about the effectiveness and safety of their products. Such trials include APSAC intervention mortality study (AIMS) (anistreplase versus placebo), Anglo-Scandinavian study of early thrombolysis (ASSET) (alteplase versus placebo) and ECSG-V (alteplase versus placebo). All these studies were successful in achieving their primary aim, but attempts to extrapolate beyond a simple demonstration of benefit and to argue for the superiority of one agent over another on the basis of percentage mortality reductions have led to much confusion.

THE AIMS STUDY

This trial compared anistreplase 30 units with placebo in patients under 70 with ECG and clinical evidence of acute infarction and a symptom duration of less than 6 hours (Fig. 3.6). All patients received heparin and warfarin, but not aspirin. For ethical reasons, a 'stopping rule' was built into the trial so that an independent monitoring group could stop the study if clear evidence of superiority of one form of treatment emerged. In the event, the stopping rule was invoked when just over 1000 patients had been entered, and the 4-week fatality rates were 12.2% in the placebo group and 6.4% in the treated group, a mortality reduction of 47% (95% confidence intervals 21–65%). A quirk of the AIMS study was that the placebo group mortality, and the percentage mortality reduction with treatment were both greater in the patients treated 3–6 hours after symptom onset than in those treated in under 3 hours. This effect has not been seen in other trials and there is no provable explanation for it, though I suspect it results from inadvertent selection bias which led to a greater inclusion of low-risk patients in the 0–3 hours group and to their exclusion from the 3–6 hours group.

THE ASSET TRIAL

This trial adopted a different philosophy as well as a different agent. It relied on clinical criteria for infarction, and deliberately included patients with normal or relatively normal electrocardiograms: these turned out to have a low mortality. Patients were randomized to placebo or to 100 mg alteplase (Fig. 3.7). Heparin was given for 24 hours, but no aspirin or long-term

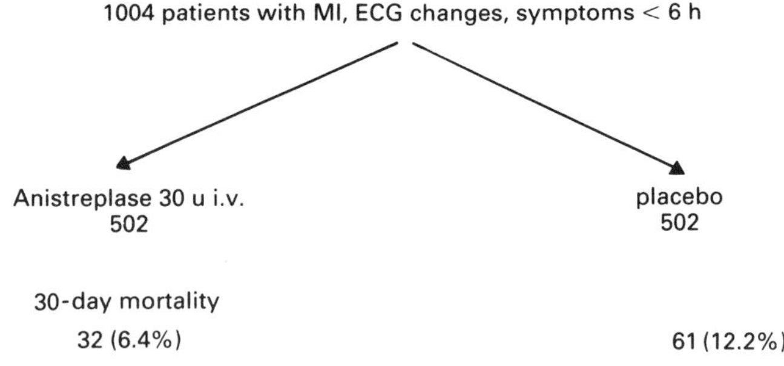

Fig. 3.6 The APSAC intervention mortality study (AIMS). (From AIMS trial Study Group (1988) *Lancet*, **i**, 545–549.)

anticoagulation was used. Mortality at 4 weeks in the placebo group was 9.8% (rising to 11.2% if low-risk patients were excluded) and in the treated group it was 7.2%, giving a relative mortality reduction of 26% (95% confidence intervals 11–39%). Simultaneously with the ASSET study, the ECSG-V trial also compared alteplase and placebo, but in a study with ostensibly more rigorous ECG criteria which *should* have led to a greater proportion of high risk patients and a higher placebo group mortality. On the contrary, the placebo group mortality in this study was extremely low at 5.8%, and although the mortality was even lower in the treated group at 2.8% the small number of events led to wide confidence intervals (relative mortality reduction 51%, 95% confidence intervals 2–67%). I strongly suspect that 'inadvertent' selection bias also operated in this study, since although it was largely conducted in district hospitals the message of the GISSI study had by this time been widely appreciated, and there were considerable pressures to divert

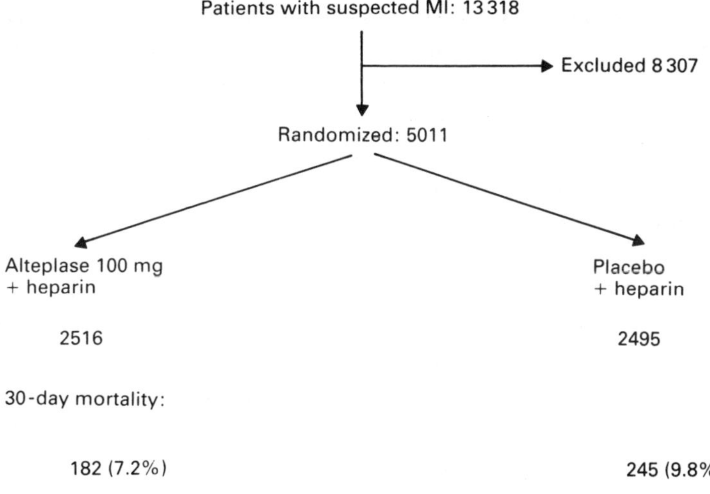

Fig. 3.7 Anglo Scandinavian trial of early thrombolysis (ASSET). (From Wilcox, O. *et al.* (1988) *Lancet*, **ii**, 525–530.)

high-risk patients away from a study which still had a placebo arm.

In summary, efforts to extract information about the relative efficacy of different agents from mortality rates in placebo-controlled trials are highly suspect. The appropriate way to secure such information is to use limited surrogate endpoint studies for preliminary screening and dose ranging, and then to go on to large scale direct comparisons such as the current GISSI-2 and ISIS-3 studies.

Which subset of patients benefit most?

Can trials be used to identify patients who appear to gain special benefit from thrombolysis, or conversely patients in whom thrombolysis is relatively ineffective? Yes, but since this inevitably involves subset analysis, the answers are less precise than those to the simpler questions the trials were designed to answer. There is general agreement (apart from the AIMS study) that early treatment gives the best results. However, there is controversy over the appropriate 'time window' during which treatment is worthwhile, with ISIS-2 suggesting significant benefit even after 12 hours, and GISSI denying it. Unfortunately we cannot go back and alter our data collection retrospectively, so we shall never know how many of the 'late entry' patients in ISIS had 'stuttering infarcts' and how many had early symptoms and then a long asymptomatic delay.

Mortality reduction is greatest among those with anterior infarction and considerable ST elevation. The ISIS-2 study (but not GISSI) also showed benefit in patients with inferior infarction and those who had previously had an infarct. These and other details are discussed further in Chapter 4. In general, since 'lack of proof of benefit' is much more common than 'proof of lack of benefit' it is good policy to be liberal rather than restrictive in interpreting the results of trials. It is tempting to design studies specifically to answer detailed questions such as the role of thrombolytic therapy in patients presenting with cardiogenic shock more than 6 hours after the onset of symptoms, but in general cardiologists have proved less able than oncologists at such investigational hairsplitting, and such studies have failed to recruit patients.

Further reading

APSAC Invention Mortality Study (AIMS) trial group (1988) Effect of intravenous APSAC on mortality after acute myocardial infarction: preliminary report of a placebo controlled clinical trial. *Lancet*, **i**, 545–549.

de Bono, D.P. (1987) Jubilee editorial: Coronary thrombolysis. *British Heart Journal*, **57**, 301–305.

Breddin, K., Ehrly, A.M., Fechler, L. *et al.* (1973) Die kurtzeit Fibrinolyse beim akuten Myocardinfarkt. *Deutsch Medizinische Wochenschrift*, **98**, 861–873.

Fletcher, A.P., Alkjaersig, N., Smyrniotis, F.E. & Sherry, S. (1958) The treatment of patients suffering from early myocardial infarction with massive and prolonged streptokinase therapy. *Transactions of the Association of American Physicians*, **71**, 287–295.

Gruppo Italiano per lo Studi della Streptochinasi nell' Infarto miocardico (GISSI) (1986) Effectiveness of intravenous thrombolytic therapy in acute myocardial infarction. *Lancet*, **i**, 397–401.

Schröder, R., Biamino, G., Leitner, E.R. *et al.* (1983) Intravenous short term infusion of streptokinase in myocardial infarction. *Circulation*, **67**, 536–548.

Second International Study of Infarct Survival Collaborative Group (ISIS-2) (1988) Randomized trial of intravenous streptokinase, oral aspirin, both or neither among 17 187 cases of suspected myocardial infarction: ISIS-2. *Lancet*, **ii**, 349–360.

The TIMI study group (1985) The thrombolysis in myocardial infarction (TIMI) trial. Phase 1 findings. *New England Journal of Medicine*, **312**, 932–936.

van de Werf, F., Ludbrook, P.A., Bergmann, S.R. *et al.* (1984) Coronary thrombolysis with tissue type plasminogen activator in patients with evolving myocardial infarction. *New England Journal of Medicine*, **310**, 609–613.

Verstraete, M., Bernard, R., Bory, M. *et al.* (1985) Randomized trial of intravenous recombinant tissue type plasminogen activator versus intravenous streptokinase in acute myocardial infarction. *Lancet*, **i**, 842–847.

Verstraete, M., Bleifeld, W., Brower, R.W. *et al.* (1985) Double blind randomized trial of intravenous recombinant tissue type plasminogen activator versus placebo in acute myocardial infarction. *Lancet*, **ii**, 965–969.

Wilcox, R.G., von der Lippe, G., Olsson, C.G., Jensen, G., Skene, A.M. & Hampton, J.R. (1988) Trial of tissue plasminogen activator for mortality reduction in acute myocardial infarction: Anglo Scandinavian Study of early thrombolysis (ASSET). *Lancet*, **ii**, 525–530.

Yusuf, S., Collins, R. & Peto, R. (1985) Intravenous and intracoronary fibrinolytic therapy in acute myocardial infarction: overview of results on mortality, reinfarction and side effects from 33 randomised controlled trials. *European Heart Journal*, **6**, 556–585.

4: Selection of Patients for Thombolysis

Patients are suitable for coronary thrombolysis if: (a) they have had a coronary thrombosis causing reversible myocardial ischaemia; and (b) the benefits of thrombolytic therapy would outweigh the risks.

Diagnosis of coronary thrombosis

In the early days of thrombolytic therapy, clinical trials insisted on rigid and stringent ECG criteria for acute myocardial ischaemia before thrombolytic therapy could be given. This was partly because thrombolysis was regarded as novel and potentially hazardous therapy, and partly because for clinical trial purposes it was necessary to select patients with a high probability of angiographic coronary occlusion. There is no doubt that these criteria (Table 4.1) based on the detection of specified amounts of ST elevation (Fig. 4.1), have a high degree of specificity. However it was always suspected that such rigid criteria would in practice exclude a large number of patients who might benefit from thrombolysis. This was confirmed in the ISIS-2 study where a group of patients in whom it was impossible to obtain definite ECG confirmation of either anterior or inferior infarction, nevertheless showed a considerable mortality, and considerable benefit from thrombolysis. However, in the ASSET study a

Table 4.1 Criteria for diagnosis of myocardial infarction used in the first two ECSG trials.

1 Chest pain of ischaemic type lasting for >30 min
2 ST segment elevation >2 mm in at least two frontal plane ECG leads *or*
3 ST elevation >3 mm in at least two chest leads (V2–V6)

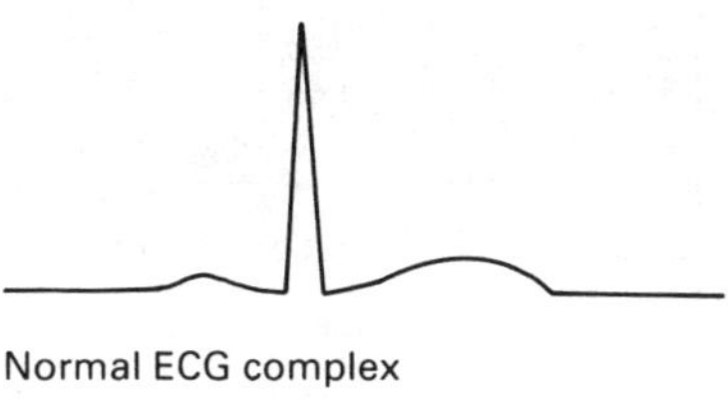

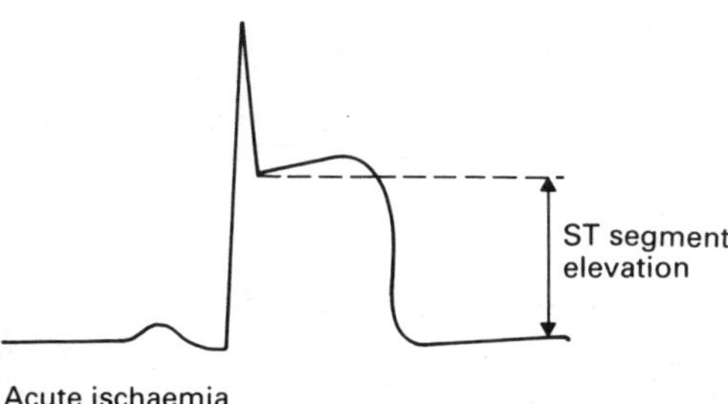

Fig. 4.1 The most striking ECG change in acute myocardial ischaemia is elevation of the ST segment.

group of patients with completely normal cardiograms had a very low mortality when allocated to placebo therapy.

The reliability of the clinical diagnosis of myocardial infarction will depend both on the experience of the clinician making the diagnosis and on the reliability of the criteria used. Multivariate analysis of clinical features at presentation in a group of patients in whom myocardial infarction was subsequently confirmed have emphasized the importance of age, male sex, severity and duration of pain, and the clinical findings of sympathetic activation (pallor, sweating), tachycardia, hypotension, a narrow pulse pressure and frequent extrasystoles. These factors have been combined in an ingenious slide rule (Ami-ri-minometer/Imi-ri-minometer, Boehringer Ingelheim) and can also be incorporated into record sheets or computer programs to assist diagnosis (Fig. 4.2).

In practical terms, a strong clinical suspicion of myocardial infarction by an experienced clinician, combined with at least some ECG evidence of acute ischaemia, are adequate grounds

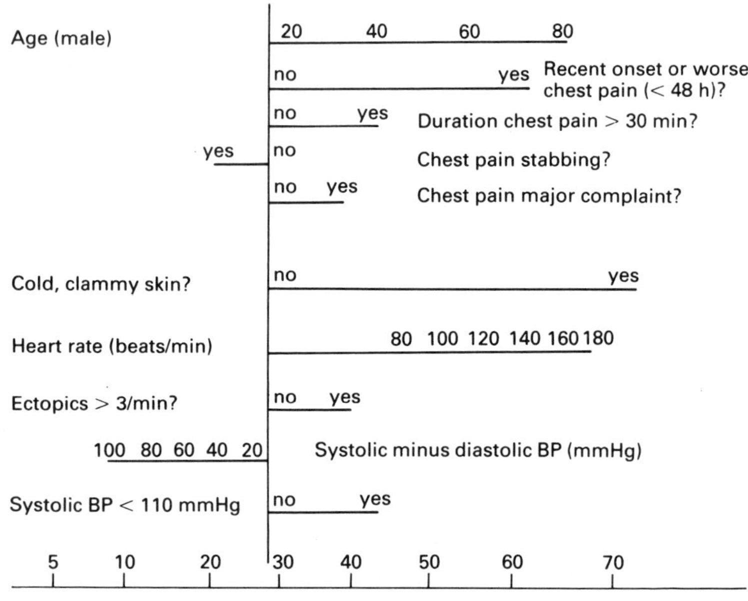

Fig. 4.2 Clinical diagnosis of myocardial infarction. Bars to the right of the centre line indicate increasing likelihood of myocardial infarction, to left decreasing likelihood. By adding up the length of bars for each feature present, the likelihood of infarction can be estimated from the scale at the bottom. (From Lubsen, J., Pool, J. & van der Does, E. (1978) *Methods of information in medicine*, **17**, 127–129.)

for initiating thrombolysis (Table 4.2). If thrombolysis is to be started before the patient has been reviewed by an experienced clinician, e.g. by ambulance crews or paramedics, then it would be prudent to insist on more stringent ECG criteria even if these exclude some patients who might have benefitted.

Duration of myocardial ischaemia

Laboratory experiments in dogs have shown that sudden, complete occlusion of a coronary artery leads to progressive irreversible damage in the area supplied by the artery, and restoration of blood flow after periods longer than 3 hours is ineffective in

Table 4.2 Consensus criteria for initiating thrombolytic therapy in suspected myocardial infarction. (Based on ASSET and ISIS-2 criteria (1989).)

1 Strong clinical suspicion of myocardial infarction based on type, severity and duration of chest pain
2 At least some ECG evidence of myocardial ischaemia or infarction
3 Absence of major contraindications

restoring function. The critical period differs in other animals because of different degrees of collateral blood flow. Clinical experience tends to support the dog model—even very short periods of coronary occlusion may cause irreversible damage, and clinical trials have failed to demonstrate preservation of left ventricular function after total ischaemic periods of greater than 4 hours. However, large scale trials using mortality rather than ventricular function as endpoints have shown worthwhile improvements in survival with thrombolytic therapy compared to placebo in patients with symptom durations as long as 6 hours (AIMS study), 9 hours (GISSI study), or even 24 hours (ISIS-2).

The most probable explanation is that clinical coronary occlusion is often intermittent, with periods of complete occlusion alternating with periods of restored flow. None of the large trials mentioned has been able to separate patients with 'stuttering' infarcts from those with 'big bang' infarcts where a major vessel is suddenly occluded and remains blocked. However the latter tend to present with more striking clinical symptoms, and probably tend to receive treatment earlier. Alternative explanations include 'conditioning' of myocardium to ischaemia by a pre-existing severe stenosis, or protection of the myocardium by collaterals. Collateral filling of the distal part of a vessel blocked by thrombus is actually very rare in the first few hours of myocardial infarction.

Site of infarct

Although overall patient mortality is approximately similar for anterior and inferior wall infarcts, the mechanisms differ. Patients with inferior wall infarcts tend to die from electrical catastrophes, often before reaching medical care, while patients with anterior wall infarction who survive to reach hospital may subsequently die from pump failure related to impaired left ventricular function. Thrombolytic therapy consistently shows improvement in left ventricular function on patients with anterior infarction, but earlier studies failed to show an improvement in patients with inferior infarction. To some extent, this was an artifact of the technique used to measure left ventricular function, and more sophisticated methods have now shown preservation of function in inferior as well as in anterior infarcts. Larger-scale mortality studies have shown that mortality is reduced in both anterior and inferior infarcts, and to proportionately the same extent. Because mortality in patients who reach hospital is higher with anterior than inferior infarcts, the *absolute* reduction in mortality (i.e. lives saved/100 patients treated) is greater for anterior infarcts. In practice, thrombolytic therapy should be offered to patients with both anterior and inferior infarcts, but in marginal cases the better prognosis in patients with inferior infarction who reach hospital may be taken into account.

Age of the patient

Age is a powerful independent risk factor in mortality from myocardial infarction: older patients are much more likely to die from an episode of infarction than younger ones. Those clinical trials which have included patients over 65, or which have had no upper age limit, have demonstrated that thrombolytic therapy markedly reduces infarct mortality in elderly patients. There is some evidence that elderly patients have a higher incidence of bleeding complications, but this is at least in part related to their tendency to have a smaller body mass and thus to receive a proportionately higher dosage of thrombolytic agent.

Contraindications to thrombolytic therapy

Contraindications to thrombolytic therapy are usually relative rather than absolute: the potential risks have to be weighed against the possible benefits. A consensus conference at the National Institute of Health in 1980 drew up a 'consensus list' of contraindications to thrombolysis which is shown in Table 4.3. This list is a useful starting point for comment and discussion.

Absolute contraindications

Active internal bleeding remains an absolute contraindication. Many cardiologists would regard a previous documented intracerebral haemorrhage or subarachnoid haemorrhage at any point in the past as a very strong, though not perhaps an absolute, contraindication. A cerebrovascular accident within the past 2 months not thought to be due to haemorrhage is a relative rather than an absolute contraindication.

Relative major contraindications

Major surgery, obstetrical delivery, organ biopsy or puncture of non-compressible vessels within 10 days, recent serious gastrointestinal bleeding and recent serious trauma continue to be major contraindications. Trauma to the head should always be considered 'serious' in the context of thrombolysis. Severe arterial

Table 4.3 Contraindications to thrombolysis. (From National Institute of Health consensus conference (1980).)

Absolute

Active internal bleeding, cerebrovascular accident within 2 months, other active intracranial process

Relative major

Major surgery, obstetrical delivery, organ biopsy or puncture of non-compressible vessels within 10 days
Recent serious gastrointestinal bleeding
Recent serious trauma
Severe arterial hypertension

Relative minor

Recent minor trauma or cardiopulmonary resuscitation
High likelihood of left heart thrombus
Bacterial endocarditis
Haemostatic defect
Pregnancy
Diabetic hemorrhagic retinopathy
Age over 75 years

hypertension is no longer considered a contraindication to thrombolytic therapy in myocardial infarction, provided it can be controlled (systolic < 180 mmHg) before treatment is started. However, prolonged or traumatic cardiac resuscitation should probably be considered a major rather than a minor contraindication.

Relative minor contraindications
A high likelihood of a left heart thrombus or bacterial endocarditis would be uncommon contraindications in the context of acute infarction. The most common 'haemostatic defects' are due to anticoagulant or aspirin therapy, and should not be regarded as contraindications to thrombolysis for myocardial infarction. There is virtually no experience with thrombolytic therapy in serious or hard-to-reverse haemostatic problems such as haemophilia, but it would be sensible to avoid it. The risk in pregnancy is mainly to the fetus from retroplacental haemorrhage, and to the mother from premature labour. Myocardial infarction in pregnancy tends to carry a poor prognosis, and thrombolysis may be justified. Diabetic *haemorrhagic* retinopathy is a relative contraindication, which really applies only to patients with proliferative retinopathy—it is unfortunate that the concept has been mistakenly extended by some to include a ban on thrombolytic therapy for all diabetics! Age over 75 years is no longer regarded as a contraindication to thrombolysis for myocardial infarction.

With these modifications, it is possible to produce an updated table of contraindications—Table 4.4.

Summary

- Consider thrombolytic therapy in:
  - Patients with definite ECG evidence of infarction.
  - Patients with a strong clinical suspicion of infarction and at least some ECG evidence of ischaemia.
  - All patients presenting within 6 hours of symptom onset.
  - Patients with longer histories but evidence of ongoing ischaemia.

Table 4.4 Current contraindications to thrombolysis in acute myocardial infarction.

Absolute
Active internal bleeding
Previous subarachnoid haemorrhage or intracerebral haemorrhage

Relative major
Major surgery, obstetrical delivery, organ biopsy or puncture of non-compressible vessels within 10 days
Recent serious gastrointestinal bleeding
Recent serious trauma, including any head injury
Cerebral infarct within 2 months
Prolonged or traumatic cardiopulmonary resuscitation

Relative minor
Recent minor trauma
Pregnancy
Diabetic hemorrhagic and proliferative retinopathy
Age over 75 years

Patients with anterior, inferior or 'unclassifiable' infarcts.
Patients of any age.

- Avoid thrombolytic therapy in patients with active internal bleeding, or who have had subarachnoid or intracerebral haemorrhage within 2 months.
- For other contraindications (Table 4.4) balance the potential benefit of thrombolysis against the risk.
- Start thrombolytic therapy as rapidly as possible!

Further reading

AIMS trial study group (1988) Effect of intravenous APSAC on mortality after acute myocardial infarction: preliminary report of a placebo controlled clinical trial. *Lancet*, **i**, 545–549.

National Institute of Health (1980) Consensus development conference: Thrombolytic therapy in thrombosis. *Annals of Internal Medicine*, **93**, 141–144.

Second International Study of Infarct Survival Collaborative Group (ISIS-2) (1988) Randomized trial of intravenous streptokinase, oral aspirin, both or neither among 17 187 cases of suspected myocardial infarction: ISIS-2. *Lancet*, **ii**, 349–360.

Wilcox, R.G., von Der Lippe, G., Olsson, C.G., Jensen, G., Skene, A.M. & Hampton, J.R. (1988) Trial of tissue plasminogen activator for mortality reduction in acute myocardial infarction: Anglo Scandinavian study of early thrombolysis (ASSET). *Lancet*, **ii**, 525–530.

5: Minimizing Delays before Thrombolytic Treatment

The importance of instituting thrombolytic therapy promptly is repeatedly emphasized in this book. A summary of ways in which delays might be reduced is given in Table 5.1. Delays before initiating treatment can be divided into delays before seeking medical help and delays between seeking help and starting therapy.

Delays before seeking medical help

Myocardial infarction can present in many ways. Sudden complete proximal occlusion of a major vessel in the absence of collaterals almost invariably causes severe pain and distress, and these patients or their companions seek help rapidly. Subtotal or intermittent coronary occlusion, however, causes pain which

Table 5.1 Ways of reducing delay to thrombolytic therapy.

Patient and family education
Encourage telephone advice-seeking
Encourage self-referral or ambulance call where appropriate
Single telephone number for admission of 'query infarct' patients
Ambulance or ambulance control to warn hospital of arrival
Direct admission to CCU/pre-CCU if possible
Fast track flagging of chest pain patients in casualty
Immediate 12-lead ECG on arrival
Reference cards with management policy and treatment details
Start treatment in casualty rather than after transfer
Regular audit and review of delays
Use simple drug regime
Consider coronary ambulance/trained ambulancemen or paramedics
Family practitioners may be best people to give thrombolysis in isolated rural areas.

may be intermittent and atypical, and is often misinterpreted as 'indigestion'. There is some evidence that the time pattern of presentation may be bimodal, with an early peak corresponding to 'big bang' infarcts, and a later one to 'continuous evolution' or stuttering infarction. There is also some evidence that it is the 'big bang' infarcts which cause the most myocardial damage, and which offer the greatest scope for benefit from thrombolysis.

In the UK, most people live in urban or semi-rural areas; it is usual to call the ambulance service for patients with sudden and dramatic symptoms, and the family practitioner for illness which seems to be less serious.

Attempts have been made to persuade patients with chest pain to call a special 'hotline' telephone number, but on evaluation this has made little objective difference to the referral pattern. Perhaps this is not surprising when physicians are notoriously tardy in diagnosing their own infarcts!

British family practitioners have been less than enthusiastic about schemes which encourage patients with minor chest pain to refer themselves to hospital. This is partly perhaps because a practitioner who encouraged self-referral might (irrationally) be regarded as in breach of his contractual duty to visit a patient on demand, but more realistically because they feel hospital services would be swamped with inappropriate self-referrals. In view of the scanty response to a 'hotline', this is arguable. The extent of public response will inevitably reflect the general level of public knowledge — as public information about the potential benefits of early presentation and treatment increase, future studies of early self referral may be more rewarding.

Delays between seeking help and the initiation of treatment

There are two models for thrombolytic treatment: either the patient can be transported as rapidly as possible to hospital and treatment started there, or treatment can be started outside hospital.

At present the vast majority of patients receive thrombolytic therapy only after arrival at hospital. For patients living in urban or semi-rural areas the delay between calling an ambulance and the patient arriving in hospital is likely to be fairly short. Time can be saved by calling the ambulance at the same time as the family practitioner, by having a single coordinating telephone number so that practitioners do not have to 'phone around' to find a hospital bed, and by warning the hospital of the arrival of a potential candidate for thrombolysis.

Studies have consistently shown a potential for unacceptable delay between arrival in hospital and the start of treatment. This is particularly troublesome if patients are delivered to a casualty or accident and emergency department rather than directly to a coronary care unit, and if an inflexible heirarchy demands serial assessment by casualty officer, junior physician and senior physician before treatment is started. In some units, delay in recording a cardiogram has been a limiting factor.

Direct delivery to the coronary care unit has sometimes been impracticable because beds are 'blocked' with patients awaiting discharge, or it is feared that patients with non-infarct chest pain would be inappropriately admitted. To some extent this can be avoided by using a 'pre-CCU'—simply equipped area adjacent to the CCU where patients can be assessed and if necessary directed elsewhere.

Management in casualty departments can be streamlined by 'flagging' record with a fast-track sticker, and by laying down simple and clear-cut rules about delegating decision making to personnel likely to be immediately available. Good intentions tend to decay with a half-life of about 6 weeks, so regular supervision and reinforcement is required. It is usually preferable to start treatment in the casualty department rather than await transfer to a ward or CCU. In a busy casualty department there are great advantages in treatments which are easy and swift to administer, and anistreplase may have an advantage over other agents in this respect.

Systems in which thrombolytic therapy is taken to the patient, rather than the patient to therapy, undoubtedly give the best opportunity for early treatment. Apart from avoiding the delay in taking the patient to hospital, they also avoid delays between arrival in hospital and starting treatment. The price to be paid is that they make much greater demands on personnel and resources.

The most effective experiences of out-of-hospital thrombolysis have so far been in the context of a dedicated coronary ambulance. This is permanently on call, and takes a physician and one or more paramedics, plus ECG equipment and a defibrillator, to the patient's bedside. Diagnosis is based on ECG and clinical criteria, and on average takes about 20 minutes. Thrombolytic therapy is then administered and the patient taken to hospital. The Jerusalem and Belfast experiences indicate that this approach is feasible, that it results in earlier thrombolysis, and that as a consequence there is (probably) improved myocardial salvage. The disadvantages are that it is necessary to have appropriately trained medical staff constantly available, and that the ambulance cannot be in two places at once.

An alternative approach is to delegate responsibility for the diagnosis of infarction and the administration of thrombolytic therapy to ambulancemen or paramedics. Various ingenious devices have been made for transmitting an ECG signal from an ambulance to base, but it is probably easier to train a paramedic to recognize the ECG features of acute infarction, and to insist that these be present before thrombolysis is started.

Another option is to rely on diagnosis and thrombolytic administration by family practitioners. A check-list for those

Table 5.2 Check-list for out-of-hospital thrombolysis by general practitioners.

1 Have you discussed and agreed a policy with local physicians/cardiologists/ambulance service?
2 Have you a functioning electrocardiogram and could you recognize ECG features of acute infarction?
3 Have you a defibrillator and can you use it?
4 Do you know the properties, storage requirements and dose schedule of your chosen thrombolytic?
5 Have you the right syringes, diluents, etc?
6 Have you access to atropine, adrenaline, opiates, glyceryltrinitrate and aspirin?

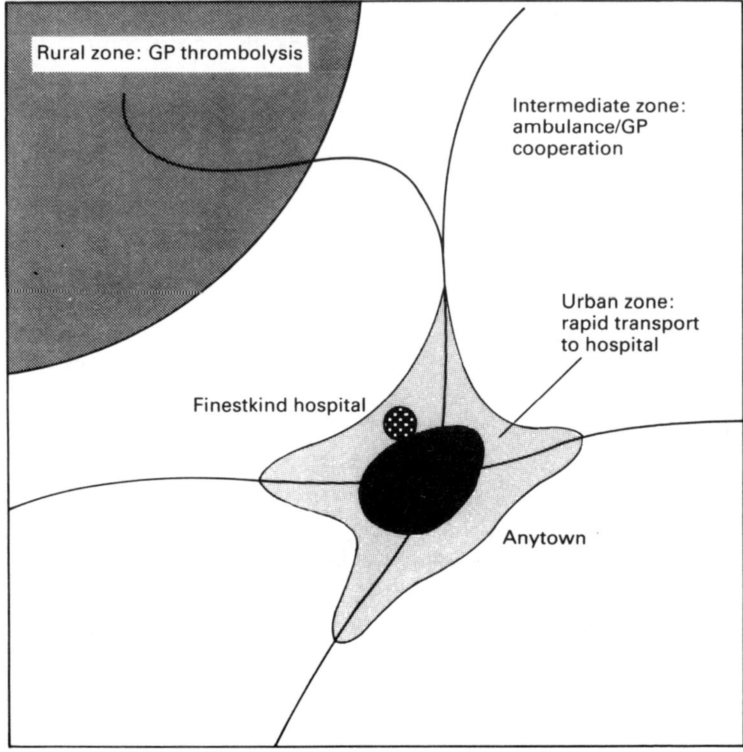

Fig. 5.1 The optimal system for early thrombolysis—based on geography.

general practitioners contemplating out-of-hospital thrombolysis is shown in Table 5.2. This is likely to be practicable, and indeed desirable, in isolated communities where the family practitioner is more likely to be available than an ambulance. Most British family practitioners in urban practices have commitments such as surgeries which restrict their instant availability, and at present the average practitioner probably sees only one or two patients a year in circumstances where it might be appropriate to start immediate thrombolytic therapy. It is likely that eventually we shall develop a system whereby the way in which thrombolytic therapy is delivered will depend on geographic zones, as shown in Fig. 5.1.

Further reading

Burns, J.M.A., Hogg, K.J., Rae, A.P., Hillis, W.S. & Dunn, F.G. (1989) Impact of a policy of direct admission to a coronary care unit on use of thrombolytic therapy. *British Heart Journal*, **61**, 322–325.

Koren, G., Weiss, A.T., Hasin, Y. *et al.* (1985) Prevention of myocardial damage in acute myocardial ischaemia by early treatment with intravenous streptokinase. *New England Journal of Medicine*, **313**, 1384–1389.

McNeill, A.J., Cunningham, S.R., Flannery, D.J. *et al.* (1989) A double blind placebo controlled study of early and late administration of recombinant tissue plasminogen activator in acute myocardial infarction. *British Heart Journal*, **61**, 316–322.

Weiss, A.T., Fine, D.G., Appelbaum, D. *et al.* (1987) Prehospital thrombolysis: a new strategy in acute myocardial infarction. *Chest*, **92**, 124–128.

6: Which Thrombolytic Agent?

Thrombolytic agents which have been shown to be effective in restoring coronary patency in acute myocardial infarction are listed in Table 6.1. Of these, alteplase, anistreplase and streptokinase currently have product licences in the UK for intravenous use in myocardial infarction. Each of these three has been shown not only to improve coronary patency, but also to reduce mortality in comparative trials against placebo.

The ideal thrombolytic agent would combine 100% efficacy with 100% safety, be easy and convenient to administer, and cost very little. It does not exist. This chapter attempts to summarize the available data about existing thrombolytics, and to assess their advantages and disadvantages. As increasing amounts of comparative data on different agents and different regimes become available, a rational choice may become easier to make, but it will continue to require subjective judgements about the relative weightings to be given to efficacy, to safety and convenience, and to cost.

Streptokinase

The relative advantages and disadvantages of streptokinase are listed in Table 6.2. There has been more clinical experience with this than with all the other agents combined.

DOSE AND ADMINISTRATION (Fig. 6.1)

A wide variety of doses have been used, but recent large trials with *intravenous* streptokinase have tended to use a 'standard' dose of 1 500 000 units administered over 60 minutes, based on an original pilot study by Schröder and colleagues. There is no particular advantage in giving a smaller dose, since streptokinase

Table 6.1 Drugs for coronary thrombolysis.

Approved name	Trade name(s)	Other names
Alteplase	Actilyse, Activase	TPA, rt-PA
Anistreplase	Eminase	APSAC, BRL26921
Saruplase		SCU-PA
Streptokinase	Kabikinase, Streptase	
Urokinase	Urokinase, Ukidan	

Table 6.2 Advantages and disadvantages of streptokinase.

Advantages	Disadvantages
Extensive experience	Risk of hypotension
Good evidence for efficacy	Not thrombus selective
Cheap	Antigenic
Stable under 25°C	Less effective on old thrombus
	Recommended dose schedule needs i.v. infusion

is relatively inexpensive and there is no evidence that a smaller dose would produce fewer bleeding complications. Indeed doses of streptokinase as small as 250 000 units can cause appreciable systemic fibrinogenolysis. A further disadvantage of low dose streptokinase is that the thrombolytic effect may be unpredictable because of pre-existing antibodies. There is some evidence that *larger* doses of streptokinase (2 000 000 or 3 000 000 units) may produce more rapid coronary reperfusion, but clinical experience with such doses is limited. It is not possible to administer the streptokinase as a bolus injection because this produces hypotension (probably as a consequence of bradykinin release) in a significant proportion of patients. There has however been satisfactory, albeit more limited, experience with its administration either as two slow intravenous injections of 750 000 units, each over 5 minutes, 20 minutes apart, or as an infusion of 1 500 000 units over 30 minutes.

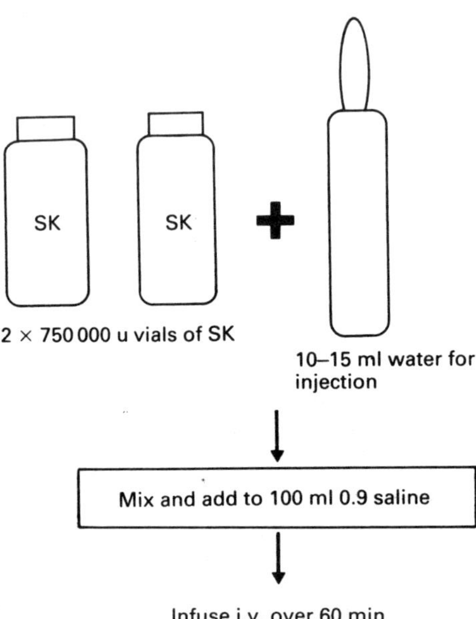

Fig. 6.1 Administration of streptokinase in acute myocardial infarction. Note that an alternative is to make up streptokinase as two injections of 750 000 u in 10 ml, each given over 5–10 min with a gap of 20 min.

Efficacy

As assessed by coronary patency. There is a difference between coronary *patency*, which is assessed by a single angiogram at a specified time after administration of the thrombolytic drug, and coronary *reperfusion*, which requires prior angiographic demonstration of coronary occlusion before treatment, followed by a second angiogram after treatment.

Reperfusion rates as high as 85% at 90 minutes have been reported with intracoronary streptokinase, but reperfusion rates with intravenous streptokinase have tended to be lower. The TIMI-1 study gave the lowest estimate, of 33% reperfusion after 90 minutes. It has been argued that streptokinase is less effective in lysing 'old' thrombus, and that the delay inherent in studies involving pre-treatment angiography make them unduly pessimistic about the efficacy of streptokinase compared to other agents. In the ECSG trial, the *patency* rate 90 minutes after initiation of intravenous streptokinase was 55%, compared with a patency rate of 70% after alteplase 0.75 mg/kg over 90 minutes. In the PRIMI trial, patency after streptokinase was 48% at 60 minutes compared with 71% after SCU-PA, and 64% at 90 minutes compared to 71% after SCU-PA.

As assessed by left ventricular function. Two moderate-sized trials have compared streptokinase (1 500 000 units) and alteplase (100 units) with respect to left ventricular function. Neither study demonstrated a significant difference in global left ventricular function, although the Plasminogen Activator Italian Multicentre Study (PAIMS) showed some advantage to alteplase in echocardiographically-assessed regional left ventricular function.

As assessed by survival. Streptokinase has not yet been compared directly with other thrombolytics in trials large enough for a realistic survival endpoint. In trials against placebo (especially the GISSI and ISIS-2 trials) survival has been better in patients treated with streptokinase than with placebo. The percentage reduction in mortality in these trials has been similar to the percentage mortality reduction observed with other agents (Table 6.3), although it is clearly very unsatisfactory to compare different trials which may have different selection criteria and standards of care.

Table 6.3 Mortality reduction and confidence intervals in trials with different thrombolytic drugs.

Trial	Agent	% mortality reduction	95% confidence intervals
GISSI	Streptokinase	18	10–28
ISIS-2	Streptokinase	22	16–28
ISIS-2	Streptokinase + aspirin	41	33–49
AIMS	Anistreplase	47	21–65
ASSET	Alteplase	26	11–39

Is streptokinase really less effective than other agents, as the patency data suggest, and the trials with LV function or mortality as endpoints simply not sensitive or extensive enough to show this? Or are the patency data irrelevant, with other effects of streptokinase such as a reduction in fibrinogen compensating for a slightly slower rate of reperfusion? Scientifically, we cannot yet distinguish between these alternatives. Practically, we know that streptokinase is effective in reducing mortality, and the onus may be on more costly agents to prove they are superior.

Safety

Streptokinase causes a profound fall in plasma fibrinogen which is usually maximal at about 6 hours and takes 12–24 hours to recover. Minor bleeding complications are frequent, but different reporting standards lead to differences in reported incidence in various trials. There is evidence that *minor* bleeding complications are more common with streptokinase than with either alteplase or SCU-PA, but the incidence of major life-threatening haemorrhage, and in particular of intracranial haemorrhage, appears to be equally uncommon (about 1%) with all available thrombolytics. Streptokinase is more likely to cause immediate hypotension than alteplase, anistreplase or SCU-PA, but this usually responds to slowing the rate of infusion. The incidence of allergic reactions and anaphylaxis (p. 64) is similar for streptokinase and anistreplase, and higher than for alteplase, urokinase or SCU-PA. There appears to be a general reluctance to use streptokinase repeatedly, though definitive evidence about its re-use is hard to come by.

Overall assessment

Cheap and effective, still the standard by which other agents are assessed. Should be used with aspirin. Side-effects definitely higher than with other agents, but no evidence that major bleeding is more common.

Alteplase

Advantages and disadvantages are summarized in Table 6.4.

Table 6.4 Advantages and disadvantages of alteplase.

Advantages	Disadvantages
More effective than streptokinase in securing coronary patency	Complex dose regime
Non-antigenic	Expensive
Thrombus selective (but little difference in major bleeding)	
Does not cause hypotension	

DOSE AND ADMINISTRATION (Fig. 6.2)
The currently recommended dose schedule for alteplase is to give 100 mg as a 10 mg bolus, 50 mg over the first hour, and 20 mg over each of the next 2 hours. The dose should be reduced to 1.5 mg/kg in patients weighing less than 67.5 kg. Alteplase has a short plasma half-life, and the rationale for a prolonged infusion is related to this, and to worries that discontinuing administration prematurely might lead to early reocclusion. Early data appeared to support this concept, but subsequent studies have been conflicting. Dose ranging studies have shown that increasing the dose from 80 to 150 mg correlates both with increasing success in reperfusion, and with earlier reperfusion.

The 150 mg dose was subsequently associated with a relatively high incidence of cerebral bleeding, and is not now recommended. Animal studies have shown that alteplase may have a persisting thrombolytic effect in thrombus for several hours after it is cleared from the circulation, and trials are in progress to examine its efficacy when given over a much shorter time period.

Efficacy

Alteplase was more effective than streptokinase at producing coronary reperfusion in the TIMI-1 study, and gave a higher patency rate than streptokinase in the ECSG-2 trial. The evidence that it produces better preservation of left ventricular function, or better survival, is at present inconclusive.

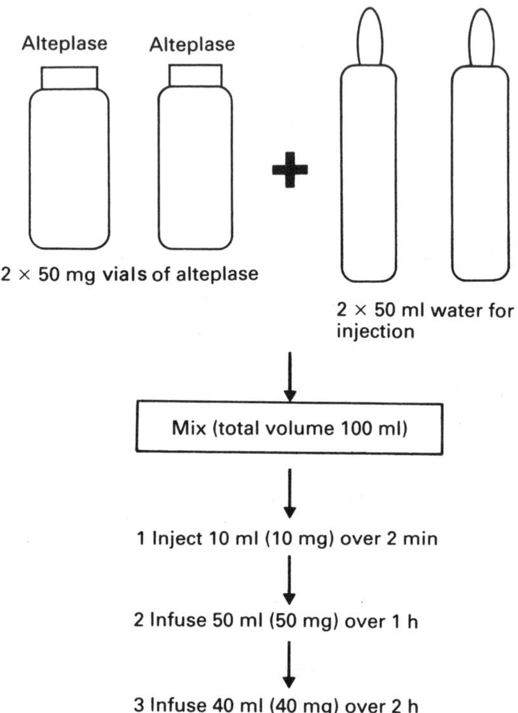

Fig. 6.2 Administration of alteplase in acute myocardial infarction. Note that if the patient weighs less than 67 kg, adjust dose to 1.5 mg/kg.

Safety

Despite its relative fibrin specificity, alteplase produces significantly more bleeding complications than placebo. Minor bleeding complications are less common than with streptokinase but the incidence of major or cerebral bleeding is similar. Anaphylaxis or allergic complications have not been reported, and hypotension during infusion is rare. Minor nausea can occur during infusion—this is probably an effect of the medium, which contains arginine, rather than of the alteplase.

Overall assessment

An effective but expensive drug. If its true impact on ventricular function and survival were to reflect its effect on coronary patency, it might be more effective than streptokinase, but this is not yet proven. Its lack of antigenicity or of significant haemodynamic side-effects are definite advantages, but disappointingly the risk of major haemorrhage is similar to streptokinase. Patients in whom there would be a particularly strong case for giving alteplase rather than streptokinase would include those who had previously been given streptokinase, patients with a strong history of anaphylaxis or allergy, patients on beta-blocker therapy, and patients with an increased bleeding risk in whom it might be necessary to terminate therapy abruptly.

Anistreplase

Advantages and disadvantages are summarized in Table 6.5.

DOSE AND ADMINISTRATION (Fig. 6.3)

Anistreplase has a relatively long plasma half-life, and immediate hypotension is less of a problem than with streptokinase, so it is usually administered intravenously as a 'slow intravenous injection' over a duration of about 5 minutes. Limited dose ranging studies have been done with intravenous anistreplase, and the largest trials have been done with a dose of 30 units which roughly corresponds to 2 000 000 units of streptokinase.

Efficacy

Intravenous anistreplase has been shown to be more effective than placebo in securing angiographic coronary patency, and the AIMS study showed a highly significant mortality reduction in patients treated with anistreplase (followed by heparin and warfarin) compared with placebo (plus heparin and warfarin).

Table 6.5 Advantages and disadvantages of anistreplase.

Advantages	Disadvantages
Effective	Expensive
Easy and quick to give	Antigenic
	Causes fall in fibrinogen
	Needs refrigerated storage

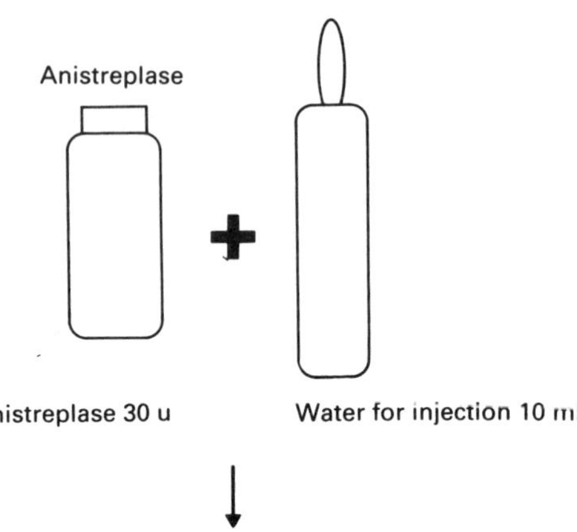

Fig. 6.3 Administration of anistreplase in acute myocardial infarction.

In a trial conducted by Anderson and colleagues, intravenous anistreplase and intracoronary streptokinase were of similar angiographic efficacy. Angiographic comparisons between anistreplase and intravenous streptokinase have been published in fragmentary fashion and are not readily interpretable. There are no convincing data comparing anistreplase with streptokinase using either left ventricular function or mortality endpoints.

Safety

The AIMS study indicated that the side-effects of intravenous anistreplase were principally haemorrhagic. The incidence of major bleeding is similar to that reported for streptokinase or alteplase. Initial hypotension is unusual, but the potential for, and probable incidence of, allergy are similar to streptokinase.

Overall assessment

This is the easiest and most convenient of the thrombolytic drugs to administer, and this may be particularly relevant for early out-of-hospital use. It is undoubtedly effective, but the absence of comparative data against other thrombolytic agents is frustrating (this should be remedied by the ISIS-3 trial). Cost is intermediate between streptokinase and alteplase.

Other agents

Urokinase and SCU-PA are both effective thrombolytic agents. Urokinase is similar to streptokinase in causing systemic fibrinogenolysis, but is non-antigenic. It has been widely used in Japan, but Western studies have been more limited, possibly because of its relatively high price. The GAU study compared alteplase (10 mg bolus, then 70 mg over 90 minutes) and urokinase 3 000 000 units over 90 minutes. Patency rates were similar (69 versus 66%) as were left ventricular function measurements. There was a non-significant trend towards a higher reinfarction rate in the alteplase group, and no difference in side-effects. SCU-PA was compared with streptokinase in the PRIMI study as described above.

There has been some interest in devising 'cocktails' of different thrombolytic agents. Initial studies suggested a possible synergism between alteplase and urokinase, with a combination of 500 000 units of urokinase and 1 mg/kg alteplase giving a similar coronary perfusion rate to 150 mg of alteplase alone and a lower re-occlusion rate. Larger scale trials are however needed.

Further reading

Streptokinase

Second International Study of Infarct Survival Collaborative Group (ISIS-2) (1988) Randomized trial of intravenous streptokinase, oral aspirin, both or neither among 17 187 cases of suspected myocardial infarction: ISIS-2. *Lancet*, **ii**, 349–360.

Alteplase

Loscalzo, J. & Braunwald, E. (1988) Tissue plasminogen activator. *New England Journal of Medicine*, **319**, 925–931.

Sobel, B.E., Collen, D. & Grossbard, E. (eds) (1987) *Tissue Plasminogen Activator in Thrombolytic Therapy*. Marcel Dekker, New York.

Wilcox, R.G., von der Lippe, G., Olsson, C.G., Jensen, G., Skene, A.M. & Hampton, J.R. (1988) Trial of tissue plasminogen activator for mortality reduction in acute myocardial infarction: Anglo Scandinavian Study of early thrombolysis (ASSET). *Lancet* **ii**, 525–530.

Anistreplase

AIMS trial study group (1988) Effect of intravenous APSAC on mortality after acute myocardial infarction: preliminary report of a placebo controlled clinical trial. *Lancet*, **i**, 545–549.

Anderson, J.L. (1988) Streptokinase and acylated streptokinase: biochemical properties and clinical effects. In Topol, E.J. (ed) *Acute Coronary Intervention.* Alan R. Liss, New York, pp. 3–24.

Anderson, J.L, Hackworthy, R.A., Sorenson, S.G., *et al.* (1989) Comparison of intravenous anistreplase (APSAC) and streptokinase in acute myocardial infarction: interim report of a randomised, double blind patency study. *Circulation*, **80**, II–420 (abstract).

Been, M., de Bono, D.P., Muir, A.L. *et al.* (1986) Clinical effects and kinetic properties of intravenous APSAC. *International Journal of Cardiology*, **11**, 53–61.

Urokinase

Mathey, D.G., Schoefer, H., Sheehan, F.H., Becher, H., Tilsner, V. & Dodge, H.T. (1985) Intravenous urokinase in acute myocardial infarction. American *Journal of Cardiology*, **55**, 878–882.

Neuhaus, K.L., Tebbe, U., Gottwik, M. *et al.* (1988) Intravenous recombinant tissue plasminogen activator (rt-PA) and urokinase in acute myocardial infarction: results of the German Activator Urokinase Study (GAUS). *Journal of the American College of Cardiology*, **12**, 581–587.

SCU-PA

PRIMI trial study group (1989) Randomized double blind trial of recombinant pro-urokinase against streptokinase in acute myocardial infarction. *Lancet*, **i**, 863–867.

Combined therapy

Topol, E.J., Califf, R.M., George, B.S. *et al.* (1988) Coronary arterial thrombolysis with combined infusion of recombinant tissue type plasminogen activator and urokinase in patients with acute myocardial infarction. *Circulation*, **77**, 1100–1107.

7: Complications of Thrombolysis – Bleeding

Abnormal bleeding is the most important complication of thrombolytic therapy. Analysis of several large scale trials of thrombolysis indicates that *minor* bleeding complications (haematomas, gingival bleeding) occur in about 25% of cases of coronary thrombolysis, *major* bleeding complications (sufficient to prolong the hospital stay) in about 5% and *life-threatening* bleeding in about 1%.

There are three principal causes of thrombolysis-related bleeding:

1 Lysis of pre-existing haemostatic thrombus, e.g. in a peptic ulcer, previous arterial puncture site, or cerebral vessel.

2 Depletion of fibrinogen and other coagulation factors (and increased levels of fibrinogen degradation products with anticoagulant effects).

3 Anticoagulation after thrombolysis.

Recent evidence suggests a fourth possible mechanism, altered platelet function as a direct effect of thrombolytic drugs in the platelet surface.

It follows that 'type 1' bleeding will be independent of the nature of the thrombolytic drug, 'type 2' bleeding will be less likely with fibrin-selective drugs and with short periods of fibrinolysis, and 'type 3' bleeding will vary with the use and level of control, of post-thrombolysis anticoagulation.

Analysis of clinical trials suggests that the incidence of major *cerebral* and *gastrointestinal* haemorrhages is relatively constant from trial to trial, and seems to be better correlated with the efficacy of the thrombolytic regime than with fibrinogen depletion. This suggests that many of these bleeds have a 'type 1' origin. Dose-ranging studies with alteplase have suggested that higher doses produce both more rapid thrombolysis *and* more cerebral bleeding. There is also some evidence that the risk of bleeding is greater in patients with a low body weight who receive a fixed dose of alteplase. There are inadequate dose ranging data to see whether a similar effect is found with streptokinase or anistreplase.

There is some evidence that cutaneous and arterial bleeds are more common with streptokinase than with alteplase, suggesting that fibrinogen depletion and its consequences may be a factor in this type of bleeding. As pointed out in Chapter 2, the degradation of circulating fibrinogen by systematically-active plasma is progressive rather than 'all or nothing', so patients who have received alteplase may have a considerable proportion of their measurable plasma 'fibrinogen' which is less haemostatically efficient than normal.

There is a clinical *impression* that patients treated with aspirin alone have fewer bleeding complications than those on heparin followed by warfarin, but proper comparative studies have not yet been done.

Spontaneous and iatrogenic bleeding

The principal sites of *spontaneous* bleeding are shown in Fig. 7.1. Invasive procedures strikingly increase the risk of bleeding, as shown in Table 7.1. Advice on avoiding bleeding associated with arterial puncture, central venous cannulation and coronary arteriography is given in Chapter 16. Serious bleeding may follow abdominal trauma or head injury, as discussed below. Sources of '*induced*' bleeding are shown in Fig. 7.2.

Cerebral bleeding

Incidence

About 1%. To put this in context, in the ISIS-2 trial the incidence of stroke was actually *lower* in patients given streptokinase, because the increased risk of cerebral bleeding was more than compensated by the reduced incidence of embolic or thrombotic stroke.

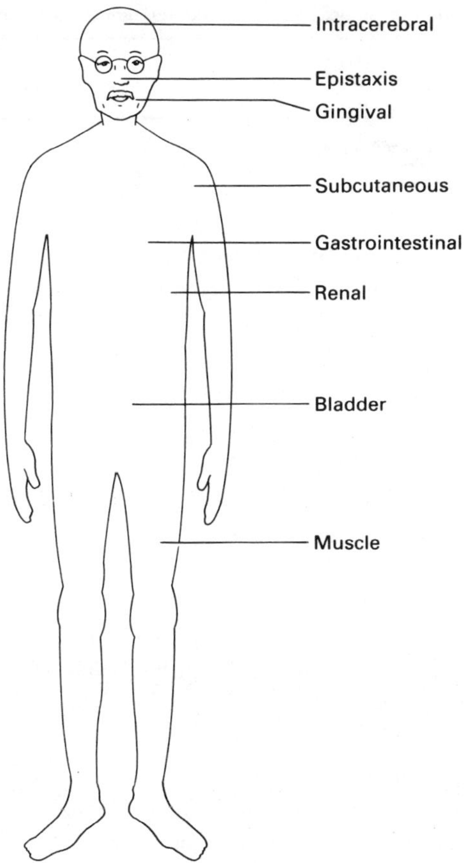

Fig. 7.1 Principal sites of spontaneous bleeding during thrombolysis.

Prevention

Avoid thrombolytic therapy in patients who have collapsed and struck their head during the presentation of the infarct—examine the head for bruises! Thrombolytic therapy is contraindicated in patients with a previous known cerebral or subarachnoid haemorrhage or cerebral arteriovenous malformation. Thrombolytic therapy in patients with a previous stroke not known to be due to haemorrhage is controversial—on balance it is probably acceptable provided the stroke occurred more than 2 months

Table 7.1 Bleeding complications and their relation to early angiography.

	Agent	Bleeding complications (%)
Trials involving early angiography		
ECSG-2	Alteplase	23
ECSG-2	Streptokinase	44
TIMI-1	Alteplase	44
TIMI-1	Streptokinase	47
ECSG-4	Alteplase	41
Trials not involving early angiography		
GISSI	Streptokinase	3.7
ISIS-2	Streptokinase + aspirin	4.5
AIMS	Anistreplase	5.4
ASSET	Alteplase	7.6
ASSET	Placebo	0.8

earlier. Hypertension is no longer regarded as a contraindication to thrombolysis provided systolic pressure can be controlled to <180 mmHg and diastolic <110 mmHg before starting therapy.

Detection

Cerebral bleeding may present either as a sudden event with headache, vomiting, obvious neurological signs and convulsions, or insidiously with increasing drowsiness and cerebral depression. Physical signs, ophthalmoscopic examination and lumbar puncture are unreliable as ways of detecting early cerebral bleeding, and the definitive investigation is computerized tomographic (CT) scanning.

Treatment

No single centre has yet had sufficient experience with thrombolysis-induced cerebral bleeding to give definitive advice, or to have compared different managements.

Neurosurgical advice should be sought immediately, and not delayed until after the CT scan. Thrombolytic therapy should be discontinued and thrombolysis reversed (Table 7.2). Support-

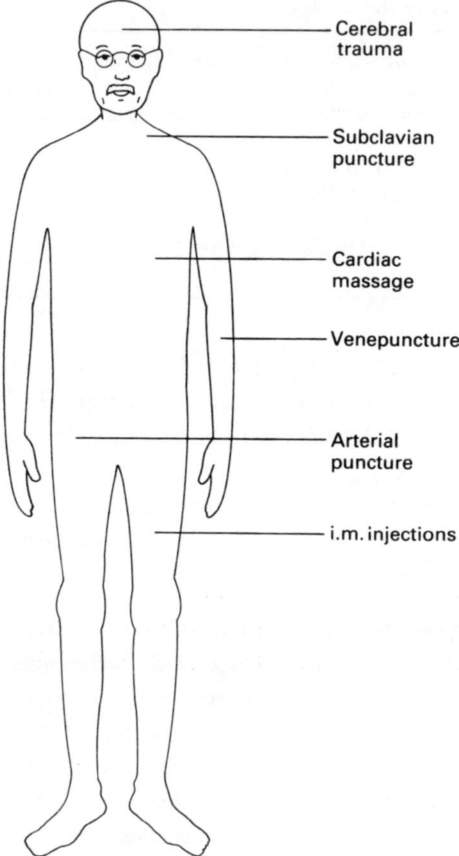

Fig. 7.2 Principal sites of iatrogenic haemorrhage during thrombolysis.

ive care of the patient should aim at preventing vomiting, extremes of hyper and hypotension, and acidosis.

Case descriptions

1 A 67-year-old woman with an inferior infarct collapsed and struck her head against a bus stop at the first onset of chest pain. She received anistreplase thrombolytic therapy 2 hours later. Four hours after that she was noticed to be drowsy and a bruise had appeared on the occiput. An emergency CT scan

Table 7.2 Reversing thrombolysis.

1 Stop infusion of thrombolytic drug and/or heparin
2 Consult with blood coagulation laboratory if possible. Take samples for measurement of fibrinogen, euglobulin lysis time, reptilase time. Cross-match blood
3 Give tranexamic acid 10 mg/kg i.v.
4 Give aprotinin (Trasylol, Bayer) 500 000 u over 10 min, then 200 000 u over 4 h
5 If fibrinogen < 1 g/l, consider giving fresh frozen plasma or fibrinogen concentrate

showed intraventricular haemorrhage and a frontal-lobe haematoma. The latter was evacuated surgically. She made a good recovery, but 2 years later she had visual impairment from belated optic atrophy.

Comment: In retrospect, thrombolytic therapy should have been avoided after the head injury. Apart from drowsiness, the physical signs were very scanty.

2 A 62-year-old man received thrombolytic therapy with anistreplase at 0900. The protocol called for heparin 1000 units/hour from 1500, but for some reason he received no heparin until 2200, when he was given 5000 units followed by 1000 units/hour. At 0200 the next morning he vomited, cried out, and rapidly developed signs of dense right hemiparesis. CT scanning showed an extensive haemorrhage in the region of the left internal capsule. Surgical evacuation of the haematoma was undertaken, but he had a severe residual hemiparesis, remained bed-bound and died 1 month later from pulmonary embolism.

Comment: It is hard to say whether or not the break of protocol over anticoagulation had any effect. The sudden and dramatic onset of symptoms contrasts with case 1.

Gastrointestinal bleeding

Incidence

Overt gastrointestinal bleeding occurs in 2–5% of patients given thrombolytic therapy for myocardial infarction. It is hard to estimate the precise incidence of occult gastrointestinal bleeding, but patients given thrombolytic therapy tend to have a greater fall in blood haemoglobin during their hospital stay than controls, and much of this is presumably due to occult gastrointestinal bleeding.

Prevention

Thrombolytic therapy is contraindicated in patients with known active peptic ulceration or oesophageal varices. Patients with a history of 'indigestion', or previous surgery for peptic ulceration, should not be excluded, but thrombolysis should be covered with a H_2 antagonist and possibly sucralfate. Haemorrhoids are not usually a contraindication to thrombolysis.

Presentation

Overt bleeding is usually upper gastrointestinal, and presents in three principal forms:

1 Early frank haematemesis. This is usually 'type 1' bleeding following the inadvertent administration of thrombolysis to a patient with an active peptic ulcer.

2 Early blood stained or 'coffee ground' vomitus. This is common in patients whose infarcts are accompanied by much nausea and vomiting, and the blood staining is largely due to multiple superficial erosions. Oral aspirin may also play a role.

3 Severe haematemesis and/or melaena late in the course of treatment (usually 24 hours or more after infarction). This is most common in severely ill patients, often with a low cardiac output, and is usually due to multiple 'stress ulcers' of stomach or duodenum.

Diagnosis

It is usually possible to decide clinically whether one is dealing with a major, life-threatening bleed or with only minor blood loss. In the first instance, resuscitation with plasma substitute and blood transfusion, cessation of thrombolysis and intravenous H_2-antagonist administration takes precedence over determining the precise source of bleeding. Once the patient is stable, upper gastrointestinal endoscopy is indicated. An emergency barium meal is a poor substitute.

Patients with continuing occult gastrointestinal blood loss after thrombolysis may need investigation for a possible colonic neoplasm.

Treatment

Patients with blood streaked or 'coffee ground' vomitus should be given an intravenous anti-emetic, an intravenous H_2-antagonist, and oral sucralfate. Blood should be cross-matched, and arrangements made for an early upper GI endoscopy. There is no need to reverse thrombolysis. Decisions about follow-up anticoagulation or aspirin therapy can be made after endoscopy.

In patients with frank haematemesis or melaena, thrombolysis should be discontinued and reversed, blood transfused, and H_2-antagonists and sucralfate given. Endoscopy should be performed as soon as the patient's condition has stabilized. Bleeding from gastric erosions or shallow ulcers will usually stop spontaneously, but a deep ulcer with a visible bleeding artery may need surgery.

Case descriptions

1 A 55-year-old man presented with an acute inferior infarct. He had an upper abdominal surgical scar, but could not give a clear account of his past medical history. He received 30 mg of anistreplase intravenously, and 30 minutes later vomited 250 ml of blood. Endoscopy revealed a previous surgical gastroenterostomy with an anastomotic ulcer. Heparin and aspirin were witheld and an H_2-antagonist given. Subsequent coronary angiography showed a patent right coronary artery and a severe left main coronary artery stenosis. He underwent coronary bypass grafting and remained well 4 years later.

2 A 65-year-old man with an anterior infarct received thrombolytic therapy with streptokinase. Despite evidence of reperfusion, he developed heart failure and arrhythmias and was not able to leave the intensive care unit. Four days after admission he had a haematemesis of 500 ml blood. He also developed melaena. He was transfused 4 units of blood and became haemodynamically stable, but then developed chest pain and ECG changes suggestive of reinfarction. Endoscopy showed multiple superficial gastric ulcers. He was treated with cimetidine and sucralfate, and eventually made a good recovery, albeit with impaired left ventricular function.

Epistaxis

This is a relatively uncommon complication. If bleeding does not respond to simple measures, the nose may need to be packed. Reversal of thrombolysis is not usually indicated, but subsequent anticoagulation may need to be deferred.

Case description

A 46-year-old woman had alteplase thrombolysis for an anterior infarct, followed by a heparin infusion. Three hours after the start of thrombolytic therapy she developed epistaxis, which continued despite local pressure and cold compresses. Heparin was discontinued and the nose packed. The pack was removed after 24 hours and aspirin given instead of heparin.

Gingival bleeding

Gingival bleeding occurs in 5–10% of patients. Anecdotally, it seems to be more common after alteplase than streptokinase. There is usually underlying periodontitis/gingivitis. Bleeding is not severe, and no special action is needed beyond reassurance, mouth washes, and eventually attention to oral hygiene.

Haematuria

Massive haematuria is rare, and in our experience frequently accompanies an unrecognized urinary tract neoplasm. Microscopic haematuria is quite common, occurring in up to 15% of patients. Transient microscopic haematuria is probably benign, but persistent or recurrent haematuria should be an indication for cystoscopy and intravenous urography. Five out of 450 patients given thrombolytic therapy in Edinburgh turned out to have urinary tract malignancies—four bladder papillomas, and one renal adinocarcinoma. Severe urinary tract bleeding should be managed in consultation with a urologist, but immediate surgery is seldom indicated.

Intra-abdominal and retroperitoneal bleeding

These are more common in patients who have sustained abdominal trauma, either as a result of a fall or during resuscitation. With intra-abdominal bleeding the patient may have vague abdominal pain, but this is not very specific. Shoulder-tip pain may occur. These patients rapidly become shocked and hypotensive. Ultrasound scanning or an abdominal top may clinch the diagnosis, and laparotomy is required. Retroperitoneal bleeding tends to be painful, with pain referred to the abdomen, back or loin. Ultrasound scanning is helpful, and the management is usually conservative (blood transfusion, analgesia, and cessation of anticoagulants).

Pericardial bleeding

There is some evidence that acute cardiac rupture may be slightly more common in patients given thrombolytic therapy. It usually presents as catastrophic hypotension and cessation of cardiac output despite inotropes, massage and, sometimes, persistence of a satisfactory cardiac rhythm. In a few patients cardiac rupture occurs in a subacute fashion, allowing echocardiographic diagnosis, pericardiocentesis, and emergency cardiac surgery.

Delayed pericardial haemorrhage is relatively uncommon, perhaps because effective thrombolysis significantly reduces the incidence of post-infarct pericarditis. A pericardial rub alone does not call for special measures or for the discontinuation of anticoagulation, but evidence of an enlarging pericardial effusion (raised JVP, enlarged cardiac shadow or the chest radiography) calls for echocardiographic monitoring, cessation of anticoagulation, and pericardiocentesis if there is evidence of incipient tamponade.

Uterine bleeding

Myocardial infarction is uncommon, but not unknown, in premenopausal women. Thrombolytic therapy has been given successfully to menstruating women, but there is a risk of increased uterine bleeding which has to be balanced against the risk of withholding thrombolysis. In pregnancy, thrombolysis carries a risk of retroplacental haemorrhage which again has to be weighed against the risks of infarction. Mechanical coronary recanalization by angioplasty may be an attractive alternative if facilities are available.

Thrombolysis after surgery

The safety of thrombolytic therapy after surgery will depend on the nature of the surgery and the length of the interval between surgery and thrombolysis. With minor surgery, a local haematoma which could be controlled by pressure might be an acceptable price to pay for thrombolysis. An arterial puncture is likely to bleed for up to 2 weeks after it has been made, and with major vascular abdominal or thoracic surgery 4 weeks would be a reasonable minimal interval. In theory, intracoronary administration of a thrombolytic would be preferable, but in practice this is often associated with substantial systemic fibrinogen depletion.

Further reading

de Bono, D.P. (1989) Problems in thrombolysis. In Julian, D., Kubler, W., Norris, R.M., Swan, H.J.C., Collen, D. & Verstraete, M. (eds) *Thrombolysis in Cardiovascular Disease.* Marcel Dekker, New York, pp. 279–292.

Erlemeier, H.-H., Zangemeister, W., Burmester, L., Schofer, J., Mathey, D.-G. & Bleifeld, W. (1989) Bleeding after thrombolysis in acute myocardial infarction. *European Heart Journal,* **10**, 16–23.

8: Other Complications of Thrombolysis

Allergy and anaphylaxis

Streptokinase and anistreplase are 'foreign' proteins which can evoke a vigorous antibody response. Alteplase, urokinase, and SCU-PA, as naturally occurring human proteins, are much less antigenic, though there is a theoretical risk that minor molecular changes resulting from *in vitro* production or storage could be recognized as foreign and give rise to antibody formation.

About 20% of the Western European adult population have detectable antibodies to streptokinase (and the streptokinase component of anistreplase), presumably from previous streptococcal exposure. Therapeutic use of streptokinase commonly leads to the appearance of detectable antibodies which appear about 7 days after treatment and persist for about 3 months.

The possible consequences of giving an antigenic drug to a patient with pre-existing antibodies are listed in Table 8.1. *Neutralization* of streptokinase activity by sera from pre-sensitized patients is actually uncommon *in vitro*, perhaps because the antibodies recognize different parts of the streptokinase molecule from those involved in its biological activity, but *in vivo* pre-existing antibodies can significantly reduce the therapeutic effect of small doses of streptokinase. The conventional dose used for coronary thrombolysis, 1.5 million units, should be large enough to overwhelm small quantities of residual antibody, but in practice there has been little reported experience, and no formal trials of efficacy, of the repeated use of streptokinase in the presence of antibodies. The repeated use of streptokinase during the period from 5 days to 3 months after its initial use is discouraged by the manufacturers. Many clinicians would prefer to use a non-antigenic drug such as alteplase for 'second time' thrombolysis

Table 8.1 Consequence of an immune response to a thrombolytic drug.

1	Neutralization of drug effect
2	Anaphylaxis
3	Early skin rashes
4	Serum-sickness like reaction
5	Vasculitis: skin lesions, nephropathy

in patients previously given streptokinase or anistreplase, irrespective of the timing of the doses.

ANAPHYLAXIS

Anaphylaxis or anaphylactic shock is potentially the most serious side-effect of repeated antigen challenge, and is due to the presence of IgE antibodies against the antigen. The onset is variable, with some patients becoming ill within seconds of the start of therapy and others having their symptoms delayed for 1–2 hours. The common features are hypotension, bronchospasm, and sometimes intense itching and an urticarial rash. There is no doubt that streptokinase or anistreplase can induce anaphylaxis, but the true incidence is difficult to assess because hypotension, although a recognized feature of anaphylaxis, may also be due to other mechanisms such as activation of the kallikrein–kinin system. The incidence of severe anaphylaxis in patients not previously given streptokinase therapeutically is probably very low (< one in 200), but mild reactions may occur in 2–3% of patients. Anaphylaxis is traditionally treated by giving a histamine H_1-antagonist, steroids to stabilize mast cells, and adrenaline to counteract both hypotension and bronchospasm (Table 8.2). In severe anaphylaxis adrenaline is the most important measure; exceptionally, patients may need intubation and respiratory support, and fluid replacement to combat inappropriate vasodilatation. There is no evidence that prophylactic use of steroids or H_1-antagonists is helpful, but these agents and adrenaline should be available whenever thrombolytic therapy with streptokinase or anistreplase is started. *Beta-blocking drugs* may make anaphylaxis more severe, and may make adrenaline ineffective as a remedy by blocking its bronchodilator effect but

Table 8.2 Treatment of anaphylaxis.

1 Discontinue drug infusion
2 Hydrocortisone 100 mg plus chlorpheniramine 10 mg i.v.
3 Adrenaline 1/1000 (1 mg/ml) 0.5 ml (0.5 mg) subcutaneously, repeated if necessary
4 Adrenaline infusion 4 μg/ml (2 ml of 1/1000 adrenaline in 500 ml saline) titrated against response
5 Intubate and ventilate if necessary

leaving its alpha (vasoconstrictor) actions unopposed. For this reason, it may be preferable to use a non-allergenic thrombolytic in patients already taking beta-blockers, and to delay beta-blocker therapy until after thrombolysis (see p. 74).

ANTIBODY-MEDIATED PLATELET AGGREGATION

This has recently been described as a potential hazard of streptokinase thrombolysis. In the patient reported, thrombus appeared to propagate despite a continuing streptokinase infusion, and streptokinase was later found to cause aggregation of platelets in the presence of the patient's plasma. This effect appears to be different from the non-antibody-dependent activation of platelets by streptokinase discussed elsewhere; data are not available to estimate its true incidence, but it would seem to be rare.

SKIN RASHES

These occur in about 5% of patients given streptokinase. Those that appear in the first 48 hours are usually macular or maculopapular multiform rashes which may fade and reappear, and sometimes itch. They are of no serious consequence and require only local treatment. They should be distinguished from the papular and sometimes purpuric lesions of vasculitis and Henoch–Schönlein purpura which are rare but important late consequences of streptokinase therapy.

VASCULITIS

This occurs in about 0.5–1% of patients given streptokinase. The onset is usually 10–20 days after treatment, and the mechanism probably involves immune complex formation between newly formed antibody and persistent streptokinase antigen. The rash is usually most prominent on the feet, and consists of raised macules, with some areas of urticaria and often of purpura. There may be fever, abdominal pain and arthralgia (Henoch–Schönlein syndrome). Microscopic haematuria and proteinuria may occur, and very occasionally glomerulonephritis may develop. Usually the condition is self-limiting and resolves without sequelae. Sometimes vasculitic lesions seem to appear in 'crops' and steroids may speed resolution. There have been isolated case reports of patients developing a progressive glomerulonephritis leading to renal failure, but this seems to be very rare. It should be remembered that other drugs which a myocardial infarct patient may receive can also cause vasculitis, including aspirin, warfarin, thiazide diuretics and antiarrhythmics.

Summary

- Streptokinase and anistreplase are antigenic and regularly induce an antibody response.
- Alteplase, urokinase and SCUPA are virtually non-antigenic in man.
- Streptokinase or anistreplase thrombolysis should not be repeated in a period 5 days to 3 months after the first dose.
- There is no restriction on repeated use of alteplase or urokinase, and they can be used after streptokinase or anistreplase.
- Anaphylaxis is rare after streptokinase or anistreplase, but adrenaline, an antihistamine and hydrocortisone should be available.
- An allergic vasculitis akin to Henoch–Schönlein purpura sometimes occurs 10–20 days after streptokinase thrombolysis. It is usually benign, but renal impairment can occur.

Reperfusion arrhythmias

In animal experiments, severe ventricular arrhythmias often follow the sudden reperfusion of viable but ischaemic myocardium. Clinically, reperfusion arrhythmias are readily recognized, particularly when coronary recanalization is done by intracoronary thrombolysis or angioplasty and the precise moment of reperfusion can be defined. However they are very seldom severe or life-threatening. The most frequent type of reperfusion arrhythmia is a short run of accelerated idioventricular rhythm at a rate usually less than 120/minute. Apart from possibly helping to identify the moment of reperfusion, this is of no significance and does not require treatment. Ventricular tachycardia or ventricular fibrillation can occur as reperfusion arrhythmias in man, but the incidence is low—of the order of 3–5%. Immediate defibrillation or cardioversion is the treatment of choice. Lignocaine may be given for up to 36 hours, but prolonged anti-arrhythmic therapy is not indicated. The incidence of *late* ventricular tachycardia, which tends to occur in patients with extensive ventricular damage, is reduced by thrombolytic therapy.

BRADYARRHYTHMIAS

These may also occur, particularly with thrombolytic treatment of inferior myocardial infarction. They usually take the form of transient sinus bradycardia or partial atrioventricular block, and seldom need treatment. Atropine is indicated if the bradycardia is prolonged. Atrioventricular block complicating inferior infarction is often abolished by coronary reperfusion, so thrombolytic therapy should *not* be withheld on account of heart block. Techniques for inserting pacing electrodes in a patient undergoing thrombolytic therapy are described in Chapter 16.

Hypotension

Hypotension after the administration of a thrombolytic drug may be a direct consequence of the thrombolytic therapy or an incidental complication of the process of myocardial infarction.

Hypotension which is due to arrhythmias is considered elsewhere. Hypotension which is not due to an arrhythmia can most conveniently be classified according to the time when it occurs.

EARLY HYPOTENSION

Early hypotension occurring during the administration of the thrombolytic drug, may be due to anaphylaxis, to activation of the vasodilator kinin system, to massive infarction or to cardiac rupture. The first two are more likely with streptokinase or anistreplase than with alteplase or urokinase. Stop giving the drug, and look for other signs of anaphylaxis (see above). If these are present, treat with steroids, antihistamine and adrenaline (Table 8.2). If not, and the hypotension is due to kinin activation, it is likely to be self-limiting and thrombolytic therapy can be resumed at a slower rate, or with a different agent. Cardiac rupture is likely to be catastrophic, and rapidly leads to circulatory standstill, sometimes with a persisting cardiac rhythm. There have been occasional reports of survival after pericardial drainage and urgent surgery, but this is exceptional. The old concept that cardiac rupture is uncommon in the first 2–3 days after infarction is wrong. Severe impairment of left ventricular function from massive infarction is a bad prognostic sign. These cases can usually be distinguished from cases of kinin activation or anaphylaxis by the absence of peripheral vasodilatation and the rapid onset of pulmonary oedema. Circulatory support with inotropes or balloon counterpulsation may be contemplated, and thrombolytic therapy should be continued, as the opening of an occluded vessel sometimes leads to a rapid restoration of ventricular function.

LATE HYPOTENSION

This is unlikely to be due to anaphylaxis, but is more likely to be due to haemorrhage. Other possible causes include right ventricular infarction, reocclusion of a previously open vessel, pericardial tamponade or the development of a ruptured papillary muscle or post infarct ventricular septal defect. If the cause is not clinically obvious, a Swan–Ganz catheter should be inserted (see Chapter 16): this will rapidly distinguish cases where rapid volume replacement is required. Bedside echocardiography may be helpful in identifying pericardial or myocardial problems.

Further reading

Bucknall, C., Darley, C., Flax, J., Vincent, R. & Chamberlain, D. Vasculitis complicating treatment with intravenous anisoylated plasminogen streptokinase activator complex in acute myocardial infarction. *British Heart Journal*, **59**, 9–11.

Hannaway, P.J. & Hopper, G.D.K. (1983) Severe anaphylaxis in drug-induced beta blockade. *New England Journal of Medicine*, **308**, 1536.

Murray, N., Lyons, J. & Chappell, M. (1988) Crescentic glomerulonephritis: a possible complication of streptokinase treatment for myocardial infarction. *British Heart Journal*, **59**, 483–485.

9: Ancillary Drugs in Thrombolytic Therapy

Aspirin

In the ISIS-2 study, aspirin alone was effective in reducing mortality after infarction, and the combination of aspirin and streptokinase was more effective than either agent alone. Unlike streptokinase, where there appeared to be a consistent trend towards better results with earlier administration, the effect of aspirin alone on mortality appeared to be virtually constant over the 24-hour admission 'window'.

Aspirin presumably works by blocking the production of thromboxane A_2 by activated platelets. This might prevent the growth of platelet thrombi, inhibit reocclusion, prevent thrombus extension or block the effects of platelet aggregation on collateral flow: data are not yet available to explain the precise mechanism. The ISIS-2 study used a specially formulated enteric-coated preparation containing 160 mg of aspirin which is not generally available—however the precise dose is unlikely to be critical. Similarly, the ISIS-2 protocol specified that the initial aspirin tablet was to be chewed in the mouth: the initial rapid absorption this produces may not be critical, but this technique might reduce gastric bleeding. Endoscopic studies in volunteers suggest that superficial gastric erosions may occur in up to 50% of subjects taking a first oral dose of conventional aspirin, but the gastrointestinal bleeding rates in the aspirin arm of the ISIS-2 study were low. It has recently been suggested that streptokinase may cause platelet activation, in which case the combination of aspirin with streptokinase thrombolysis may be particularly important. All of the studies on thrombolysis with alteplase, with the exception of the initial ECSG trials (ECSG-1 and 2) and ASSET, have included aspirin, and there are no data on whether or not it has an additional effect similar to that observed with streptokinase. Many of the European studies have given the initial dose of aspirin intravenously in an attempt to avoid gastric bleeding, but parenteral aspirin preparations are not available in the UK. Conversely, trials of anistreplase have tended to use heparin and warfarin anticoagulation but not aspirin. A trial comparing aspirin with heparin/warfarin anticoagulation after anistreplase is currently in progress.

The present consensus favours giving aspirin to all patients receiving thrombolytic therapy, in the form of oral aspirin 150–300 mg daily. The first dose should be given as soon as possible (in case it should subsequently be overlooked) and aspirin continued for at least 1 month.

Anticoagulants

In the early days of streptokinase therapy the importance of follow-up anticoagulation was emphasized, partly because the endothelium-denuded area after lysis of a thrombus was thought to provide a substratum for further thrombosis, and partly because any thrombus formed after discontinuation of streptokinase was likely to be deficient in plasminogen and therefore particularly hard to disperse. There were numerous anecdotal reports of early rethrombosis apparently related to the inadvertent or premature withdrawal of anticoagulation. On the other hand, both GISSI and ISIS-2 trials showed that thrombolysis could be effective without formal anticoagulation. Both these studies used streptokinase, which produces an anticoagulant diathesis for up to 24 hours after administration as a consequence of fibrinogen depletion and circulating fibrin degradation products with anticoagulant activity. There have been no true comparative studies of intravenous heparin versus no heparin after streptokinase, but the ISIS-3 study will look at the effects of subcutaneous heparin.

Patients receiving alteplase thrombolysis might be more susceptible to rethrombosis in that there is less fibrinogen depletion and there are fewer circulating fibrin degradation products. Most studies of alteplase thrombolysis have given up to 5 days of intravenous heparin after the alteplase. A current European cooperative study group trial is examining intravenous heparin versus heparin placebo after alteplase.

There is no doubt that prolonged intravenous heparin therapy is associated with an appreciable morbidity from haemorrhage: usually subcutaneous, but occasionally gastrointestinal or retroperitoneal. Opinions differ on whether to use a standard heparin regime (usually 1000 units/hour, or 800 units/hour in patients weighing under 60 kgs) or to titrate the dose according to some haemostatic measurement. The most commonly used is the activated partial thromboplastin time (APTT), but some use the thrombin coagulation time (TCT). In either case, the aim is to prolong the coagulation time to approximately twice normal. The regime the author has used in approximately 400 cases is to start heparin at 1000 units/hour without a loading dose 6 hours after administration of a thrombolytic agent. The heparin dose is titrated using the thrombin coagulation time twice daily (or more often). Oral warfarin is started at the same time as heparin, and the heparin is discontinued when the prothrombin time ratio (INR) exceeds 2.0.

It is impossible at present to give a consensus view on the use of heparin anticoagulation after thrombolysis. There is an increasing and understandable tendency, after ISIS-2, to omit heparin and warfarin altogether and simply to give aspirin. Current trials will help clarify the situation.

Coumadin (warfarin) anticoagulation in myocardial infarction has a similarly long history and a frustrating lack of definitive data. The inconclusive results of the Medical Research Council and Veterans Administration trials in the 1960s led to a rapid abandonment of 'routine' anticoagulation in the USA and the UK, but not on the European continent. The 'Sixty Plus Reinfarction Study' trial in the Netherlands suggested that patients given coumadins after infarction who then had them withdrawn had a higher reinfarction rate than those in whom they were continued. A number of 'overviews' have suggested possible benefit from coumadin anticoagulation. There are no comparative data on warfarin administration versus aspirin or placebo after myocardial infarction treated with thrombolytic therapy, although a heparin/warfarin regime appears to have been highly successful in the 'AIMS' study. A trial of heparin/warfarin versus aspirin after anistreplase thrombolysis is in progress. Again, it is impossible to give a consensus view, but if aspirin alone were shown to be as effective, or almost as effective, as heparin/warfarin it would undoubtedly be preferred. Patients who sustain extensive infarcts, particularly with anterior aneurysm formation and/or intraventricular thrombus demonstrable on echocardiography form a distinct group, and there is general agreement that they should be anticoagulated.

Beta-blockers

The beneficial effects of oral beta-blockers started within the first week after infarction are well-established and should form part of routine treatment for all myocardial infarction patients. The ISIS-1 study established a small but definite benefit from immediate intravenous beta-blocker (atenolol) therapy, which it has been suggested is almost entirely due to a reduction in the incidence of early cardiac rupture. Side-effects of early intravenous beta-blockade include hypotension and bradycardia, which may also occur when thrombolytic therapy (particularly with streptokinase) is given. It may be prudent, therefore, to be selective about the administration of early intravenous beta-blockade, and reserve it for patients with inappropriate hypertension or tachycardia after the thrombolytic drug has been given.

Nitrates

Nitrates are the pharmacological equivalent of the natural 'endothelial-derived relaxing factor' nitric oxide. In the context of acute myocardial infarction, they may act: (a) on the occluded vessel to counteract spasm and relieve vasoconstriction mediated by thrombin and platelet activation products; and (b) on vessels elsewhere in the body to reduce preload, and to some extent afterload, on the heart.

There is experimental evidence that spasm plays a part in facilitating thrombotic coronary occlusion, and nitrates have been shown in man to help maintain vessel patency during and after streptokinase infusion. A retrospective study of data in the European cooperative study group trials showed that prior nitrate administration was a significant independent factor in favour of coronary patency after thrombolysis with alteplase. An overview of a number of trials examining the effect of (intravenous) nitrates on survival after myocardial infarction (not specifically in the context of thrombolysis) indicates a probable improvement in survival of about 20%. The main *disadvantages* of the early use of nitrates are a tendency to hypotension, and the potential technical problems of combining an infusion of nitrates with an infusion of thrombolytic drug. A definitive clinical trial would involve giving every patient with acute infarction thrombolytic therapy (perhaps as a single injection of anistreplase) and then randomizing patients to receive either intravenous nitrate or placebo, but such a trial has not yet been done. In the meanwhile, a reasonable consensus policy would be to give all patients eligible for thrombolytic therapy sublingual nitrate (e.g. as two puffs of a sublingual spray), and to reserve intravenous nitrates (e.g. glyceryltrinitrate 2–10 mg/hour by slow intravenous infusion) for patients with persisting ischaemic pain or features of left heart failure.

Angiotensin converting enzyme (ACE) inhibitors

ACE inhibitors have an established role in the treatment of chronic cardiac failure. There is some recent evidence that their use in patients with anterior myocardial infarcts may help to prevent 'infarct expansion'—the tendency, especially after anterior infarction, for the damaged myocardium to stretch into an aneurysm-like sac which interferes with normal myocardial contraction. There is as yet no evidence that their prophylactic use in patients without heart failure improves survival.

Further reading

Aspirin

Second International Study of Infarct Survival (ISIS-2) Collaborative Group (1988) Randomized trial of intravenous streptokinase, oral aspirin, both or neither among 17 187 cases of suspected myocardial infarction. *Lancet*, **ii**, 349–360.

Beta-blockers

ISIS-1 Collaborative Group (1988) Mechanisms for the early mortality reduction produced by beta-blockade started early in myocardial infarction *Lancet*, **i**, 921–922.

Nitrates

Yusuf, S., Collins, R., MacMahon, S. & Peto, R. (1988) Effect of intravenous nitrates on mortality in acute myocardial infarction: an overview of the randomized trials. *Lancet*, **i**, 1088–1092.

ACE inhibitors

Pfeffer, M., Lamas, G.A., Vaughan, D.E. & Parisi, A.F. (1988) Effect of captopril on progressive ventricular dilatation after anterior myocardial infarction. *New England Journal of Medicine*, **319**, 80–85.

10: Angioplasty and Coronary Bypass Grafting

The introduction of intracoronary thrombolysis was rapidly followed by the realization that despite restoring coronary patency, thrombolysis frequently left a residual coronary stenosis. As a rough estimate, approximately 70% of infarct-related segments rendered patent after thrombolysis will have a residual diameter stenosis of 70% or more. These 'short segment' stenoses frequently have an appearance inviting angioplasty. Early uncontrolled experience with combined thrombolysis and angioplasty was encouraging, and subgroup analysis of the Netherlands Inter-University Study Group trial also appeared to show benefit in those patients who had had combined thrombolysis and PTCA.

The relation between angioplasty and thrombolysis can be considered as a series of questions (Table 10.1).

Should thrombolysis be followed by immediate angioplasty?

This has been examined in a number of controlled trials, particularly by the ECSG and TAMI (Thrombolysis in Acute Myocardial Infarction) groups. In the ECSG trial, which was designed to reproduce the conditions of the 'angioplasty' subset of the Netherlands inter-university trial, patients were given an intravenous infusion of alteplase and then randomized to 'intervention' or 'conservative' treatment groups.

Table 10.1 Questions about PTCA/CABG after thrombolysis.

1	Should thrombolysis be followed by immediate angioplasty?
2	Should thrombolysis be followed by delayed elective PTCA?
3	What is the role of symptom-led PTCA or CABG after thrombolysis?

In the 'intervention' group, patients were taken as rapidly as possible to the catheter laboratory and coronary angiography performed. Patients with a patent but stenosed vessel, underwent immediate angioplasty; patients with an occluded vessel had it recanalized mechanically (by poking with a guidewire) followed by angioplasty. Despite a high technical success rate for angioplasty, there was no overall benefit in terms of infarct size, left ventricular function, or survival, while complication rates (principally bleeding) were higher in the 'intervention' group. The discharge angiography showed a higher incidence of complete occlusion of the infarct related vessel in the 'intervention' group, as a consequence of subsequent reocclusion after angioplasty. If these cases are excluded, then there is slightly better preservation of left ventricular function in patients who have had angioplasty.

The TAMI and TIMI-2 trials were broadly similar in design to the ECSG study, but allowed rather more latitude to the operator in deciding, on the angiographic appearances, whether to perform angioplasty or not. Again, there was no evidence that immediate elective angioplasty confirmed benefit. A feature of both studies was that patients in the 'conservative' group could have angioplasty if this was indicated for persisting pain or threatened re-occlusion — so they should be considered as trials of thrombolysis and immediate elective PTCA versus thrombolysis and symptom-led PTCA.

Should thrombolysis be followed by delayed elective PTCA?

There are important logistic reasons why immediate angioplasty after thrombolysis is frequently impracticable, and simultaneously with the 'immediate angioplasty' trials others were set up to evaluate 'delayed elective' angioplasty after thrombolysis. These include the TIMI-2B trial (USA) using alteplase, and the SWIFT (Should We Intervene Following Thrombolysis) trial (UK) using anistreplase. The TIMI-2B study showed no benefit from delayed elective angioplasty compared with symptom-led angioplasty. The SWIFT study is presently being analysed.

What is the role of symptom-led PTCA or CABG after thrombolysis?

This can be divided into two parts. First, the role of PTCA/CABG in patients who develop rest pain or pain on minimal exertion after thrombolysis, and second, the role of follow-up exercise testing and angiography in selecting less severely symptomatic patients for intervention.

Patients who develop rest pain or pain on minimal exertion in the days immediately following thrombolytic therapy are at risk of early reocclusion, and almost invariably have a severe residual coronary stenosis. It is policy in our unit to treat these patients with heparin and intravenous glyceryl trinitrate, and to transfer them as rapidly as possible to the cardiac catheter laboratory for angiography and, usually, PTCA. The case for giving a second dose of thrombolytic agent under these circumstances is arguable: if the patient does not have persisting ST elevation or symptoms suggesting reinfarction, it is probably not necessary, but if there is likely to be a prolonged delay, or reinfarction seems imminent then a second dose should be given. It is safe to give a second dose of streptokinase or anistreplase within 1 week of the first dose; if the delay is longer a non-antigenic drug such as alteplase is preferable.

Patients who do not experience rest pain or pain on minimal exertion after thrombolysis should have an exercise tolerance test to evaluate residual ischaemia (see Chapter 11) and a decision can then be made on whether or not to proceed to angiography. The choice of PTCA or CABG as definitive treatment in these patients is based on the coronary anatomy, and our policy is to attempt to complete a revascularization as soon as possible. In selected cases, usually because of factors such as age or intercurrent illness, a more conservative approach directed towards the 'culprit lesion' is adopted.

In the author's unit, approximately 25% of patients undergoing thrombolytic therapy go on to 'symptom-led' intervention in the form of PTCA or CABG in the first year after presentation. Approximately equal numbers underwent angioplasty and coronary bypass grafting. Similar figures have been reported from

Belfast. In the TIMI-2B study 16% of patients allocated to a conservative and symptom-led approach underwent PTCA or CABG within 6 weeks of their infarct.

Summary

- Trials have failed to show any overall benefit from a policy of immediate elective angioplasty following thrombolysis.
- There is no evidence that selective angiography and angioplasty a few days after thrombolysis is any better than a policy of symptom-led investigation and intervention.
- About 25% of patients who have thrombolytic therapy may require some form of operative treatment (PTCA or CABG) for symptoms during the first year after presentation.

Further reading

Erbel, R., Pop, T., Diefenbach, C. & Meyer, J. (1989) Long term results of thrombolytic therapy with and without percutaneous transluminal coronary angioplasty. *Journal of the American College of Cardiology*, **14/2**, 276–285.

Simoons, M.L., Arnold, A.E.R., Betriu, A. *et al.* (1988) Thrombolysis with tissue plasminogen activator in acute myocardial infarction: no additional benefit from immediate percutaneous angioplasty. *Lancet*, **i**, 197–202.

TIMI Study Group (1989) Comparison of invasive and conservative strategies after treatment with intravenous tissue plasminogen activator in myocardial infarction: results of the Thrombolysis in Myocardial Infarction (TIMI) phase II trial. *New England Journal of Medicine,* **320**, 618–626.

11: Follow-up and Rehabilitation after Thrombolysis

Follow-up and rehabilitation after myocardial infarction treated with thrombolytic therapy essentially follows the standard format for post-infarction follow-up summarized in Table 11.1. Specific instances where post-thrombolysis patients may differ are summarized in Table 11.2.

The improved preservation of left ventricular function and reduction in pericarditis and late arrhythmias after successful thrombolysis helps to accelerate recovery. Care is needed however to identify patients with residual or recurrent ischaemia who may need angiography and either PTCA or coronary grafting.

Table 11.1 Follow-up after myocardial infarction.

0–24 h	Watch for arrhythmias, failure, more ischaemia
24–48 h	As above, sit out of bed
2–7 days	Gradual mobilization Watch for residual/recurrent ischaemia Rx beta blocker, aspirin, ?ACE inhibitor Assess need for other medication Start counselling Plan rehabilitation
7–9 days	Uncomplicated patients go home
4 weeks	Reassess clinical status, progress of rehabilitation Exercise test Review need for angiography
3, 6, 12 months	Family practitioner to monitor rate of rehabilitation Check lipids at 3 months Re-refer if necessary

Table 11.2 Special points after thrombolysis.

0–48 h	Arrhythmias, failure less common Watch for ischaemia Watch for haemorrhage
2–7 days	Stabilize anticoagulants if used Some patients may be suitable for early (3–4 day) discharge Low threshold for angiography if ischaemia recurs
7–9 days	Issue card indicating which thrombolytic used
4 weeks +	15–30% of post-thrombolysis patients may come to PTCA/coronary grafting in 1 year

Recurrent ischaemia

Recurrent ischaemia may present either as rest pain or as angina of effort. Its management is summarized in Fig. 11.1. Rest pain should be treated in the first instance with nitrates, preferably as an intravenous infusion (glyceryl trinitrate infusion 10–25 μg/minute). The ECG may show new ST segment changes, but these can sometimes be hard to distinguish against an underlying infarct pattern. A rise in plasma creatine kinase is usually reliable evidence of reinfarction: it is best appreciated using paired blood samples, the first taken immediately and the second, 6 hours later. Arrangements should be made for coronary angiography as soon as possible; urgency is increased if the recurrent pain is severe or persistent. Most patients who develop recurrent rest pain after thrombolytic therapy have an isolated, tight coronary stenosis in a patent infarct related vessel, and respond well to angioplasty. If angiography shows complete occlusion, an attempt can be made at mechanical recanalization by probing with a guide wire, followed by angioplasty. If the patient has multivessel coronary disease it is usual to treat the 'culprit lesion' in the infarct related vessel, and to defer further angioplasty to a later date.

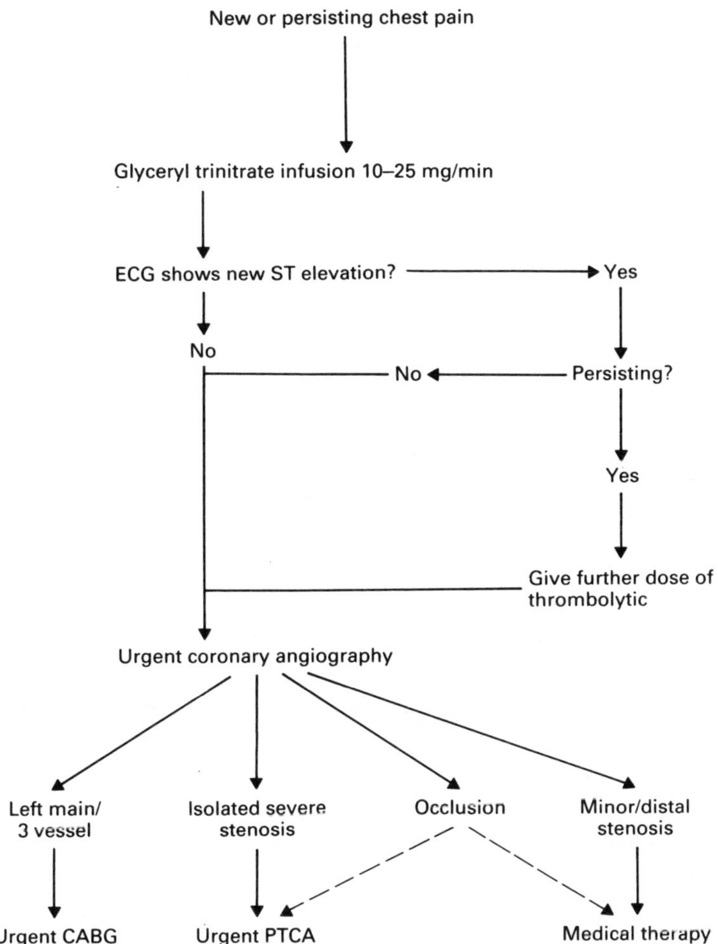

Fig. 11.1 Management of recurrent ischaemia after thrombolysis.

Occasionally a patient will have a severe proximal lesion which is not suitable for angioplasty—this is often accompanied by multivessel disease. These patients may be suitable for immediate coronary artery grafting. Provided left ventricular function is good the results of early post thrombolysis coronary bypass grafting are excellent. It is usually best to wait for

24 hours after administering thrombolytic therapy to allow coagulation to recover before surgery, and in patients given streptokinase or anistreplase it may be necessary to give fresh frozen plasma. There may be some excess bleeding associated with aspirin therapy.

If angiography shows only a stenosis in a distal or minor vessel, it is reasonable to proceed with conservative treatment.

Angina of effort, whether spontaneous or discovered on formal exercise testing, is also an indication for angiography—albeit a less urgent one. There is general agreement that patients who have had thrombolytic treatment for myocardial infarction should have an exercise test, but there is argument about the pros and cons of early submaximal testing versus maximal effort testing at about 1 month after hospital discharge. Ideally, both should be done, but this often presents logistic difficulties. A maximal test at 1 month is preferable, with a low threshold for earlier investigation, or angiography without effort testing, if clinically indicated. There is obviously little point in attempting a stress test in patients with rest pain, angina on minimal exertion, or cardiac failure.

Other tests which may have a role in the follow-up of patients with myocardial infarction are radionuclide ventriculography and echocardiography.

RADIONUCLIDE VENTRICULOGRAPHY

This provides information which can be used to identify the likely prognosis: patients with poor left ventricular function have a higher 1 year mortality. At present, the data used to define the relationship between left ventricular function and prognosis are those which were collected before the thrombolytic era: a similar relationship in post-thrombolysis patients is likely, but it is possible overall prognosis might be better.

ECHOCARDIOGRAPHY

This is less easy to quantitate than radionuclide ventriculography, but is capable of detecting locally-impaired left ventricular function and aneurysms. It may be particularly useful in identifying patients who would be particularly helped by long-term anti-coagulation (to prevent embolism from left ventricular thrombus) or long-term angiotensin converting enzyme inhibitor therapy (to prevent progressive left ventricular dilatation).

The roles of anticoagulants, aspirin and beta-blockers have already been discussed (see p. 71).

AFTER-HOSPITAL CARE

In the UK, most patients leave hospital 7–9 days after acute myocardial infarction. By this stage they are likely to be mobile around the hospital ward, free of pain and free of cardiac failure. The diagnosis of myocardial infarction and its implications will have been discussed, and a suitable programme of physical and psychological rehabilitation planned and organized. The supervision of further recovery will largely be in the hands of the family doctor, to whom full information should be given. It may be helpful to use a standard information sheet (Table 11.3). The patient and family doctor must be told that thrombolytic therapy has been given, and the name of the agent used (some manufacturers produce 'credit card' sized information cards). The date and time of the follow-up appointment should be specified, and it is important to clarify the mechanism for seeking advice if problems should arise.

A follow-up appointment about a month after hospital discharge is very useful. Apart from assessing clinical progress and complications such as post-infarct angina, this is often a better time for discussion about future work options, etc. A maximal exercise test may be done at this stage; and fasting glucose and plasma lipids should be checked—despite the continuing lack of convincing evidence for effective secondary prevention of infarction by lipid lowering drugs there is increasing consensus that correcting hyperlipidaemia improves the outcome of coronary artery surgery. Family screening may also be appropriate. A specimen check list for the 1 month follow-up is shown in Table 11.4. The author's practice is to return the majority of patients to the care of their family doctor after the 1 month follow-up

Table 11.3 Information to family practitioner at discharge.

To: Dr Jekyll Health Centre Sometown	Re: Joe Bloggs 39 Step Street Sometown Date of Birth: 05/08/45 Hospital number: 050845M
Admitted 03/03/89	Discharged 10/03/89
Consultant:	Prof. Bigcheese
Diagnosis:	Acute anterior myocardial infarction
Treatment in hospital:	Thrombolytic therapy with streptokinase 1 500 000 u
Complications:	None
Treatment at discharge:	Timolol 5 mg b.d., continue for 1 year; aspirin 150 mg daily, continue for 1 year
Follow-up:	Exercise test 12/04/89, clinic 12/04/89. Rehabilitation group Thursday evenings for 6 weeks
Information to patient:	Told he has had a heart attack, advised to stop smoking, given British Heart Foundation booklet
Comment:	Good recovery, clinical course suggested reperfusion
	Yours sincerely,
	A. Goodlad, House Officer

visit, with arrangements for re-referral in the event of any late complications or new events.

Published data on the natural history of post-myocardial infarct patients treated with thrombolytic therapy consistently indicates that the survival benefit apparent at 1 month persists at 1 year. 'Events' such as reinfarction, PTCA or coronary graft surgery are most common in the first few weeks after the initial infarct.

Table 11.4 Check-list for 1 month follow-up.

Symptoms
Chest pain?
Dyspnoea?
Other?
Examination
Heart failure?
Murmurs?
BP?
Rehabilitation
Exercise level?
Plans for return to work?
Family life?
Driving?
Tests
Exercise test?
Radionuclide ventriculogram?
Echocardiogram?
Check lipids?
Do family need lipid screen?

Summary

- The basic pattern of follow-up after myocardial infarction treated with thrombolytic drugs is similar to that established before the advent of thrombolytic treatment.
- Better preservation of left ventricular function may enable recovery to be accelerated.
- Persistent or recurrent ischaemia is an indication for angiography with a view to angioplasty or coronary artery grafting.
- Exercise stress testing is useful both for identifying and quantitating ischaemia and for indicating to patients a 'safe' level of activity.
- Data are presently lacking on whether the long-term use of aspirin or anticoagulants improves outcome and reduces the risk or reinfarction. Our present policy is to continue aspirin for 1 year.

Further reading

Campeau, L., Enjalbert, M., Lesperance, J. *et al.* (1984) The relationship of risk factors to the development of atherosclerosis in saphenous vein by-pass grafts and the progression of disease in the native circulation. *New England Journal of Medicine*, **311**, 1329–1331.

de Bono, D.P., McAreavey, D., Been, M. & Peterson, H. (1988) Long term follow up after coronary thrombolysis: the Edinburgh experience. In de Groot, C. (ed) *Hyperlipidaemia and Atherosclerosis*. Academic Press, New York, pp. 175–184.

Peart, I., Odemuniyiwa, O., Albers, C. *et al.* (1989) Exercise testing soon after myocardial infarction: its relation to course and outcome at one year in patients aged less than 55 years. *British Heart Journal*, **61**, 231–237.

12: How to do it—Practical Examples

A summary flow-chart of the immediate management of myocardial infarction using thrombolytic therapy is shown in Fig. 12.1. The rest of this chapter attempts to illustrate some of the points raised in earlier chapters by reference to some practical examples. Needless to say, there is no such person as a 'typical' patient, and everyone needs to be assessed and treated individually.

Example 1

Mr J.C., aged 46, is brought into a hospital casualty department at 0830. He had developed severe chest pain at home at 0745 and, after a telephone discussion with the family doctor, his wife telephoned directly for an ambulance.

The ambulance service has notified the casualty department of the impending arrival of a patient with chest pain, and as soon as he arrives his record is 'flagged' for fast track medical care. At 0835 a 12-lead ECG is being recorded, and he is seen by a casualty physician. On examination, he is pale and vasoconstricted, pulse 90/minute, BP 105/172, quiet heart sounds, clear chest. The ECG shows sinus rhythm with ST segment elevation in leads V2–V4. He has had no recent surgery or injury, has never previously received streptokinase, and is on no medication. There is nothing in the history to suggest peptic ulceration or subarachnoid haemorrhage. At 0840 he is given two puffs of sublingual GTN spray and an aspirin to chew. At 0845 an intravenous cannula is inserted and he is given 10 mg morphine plus 50 mg cyclizine. Blood is drawn for haemoglobin, wbc, platelets, fibrinogen, electrolytes, cholesterol and blood grouping. At 0850 an infusion of 1 500 000 streptokinase (2 ×

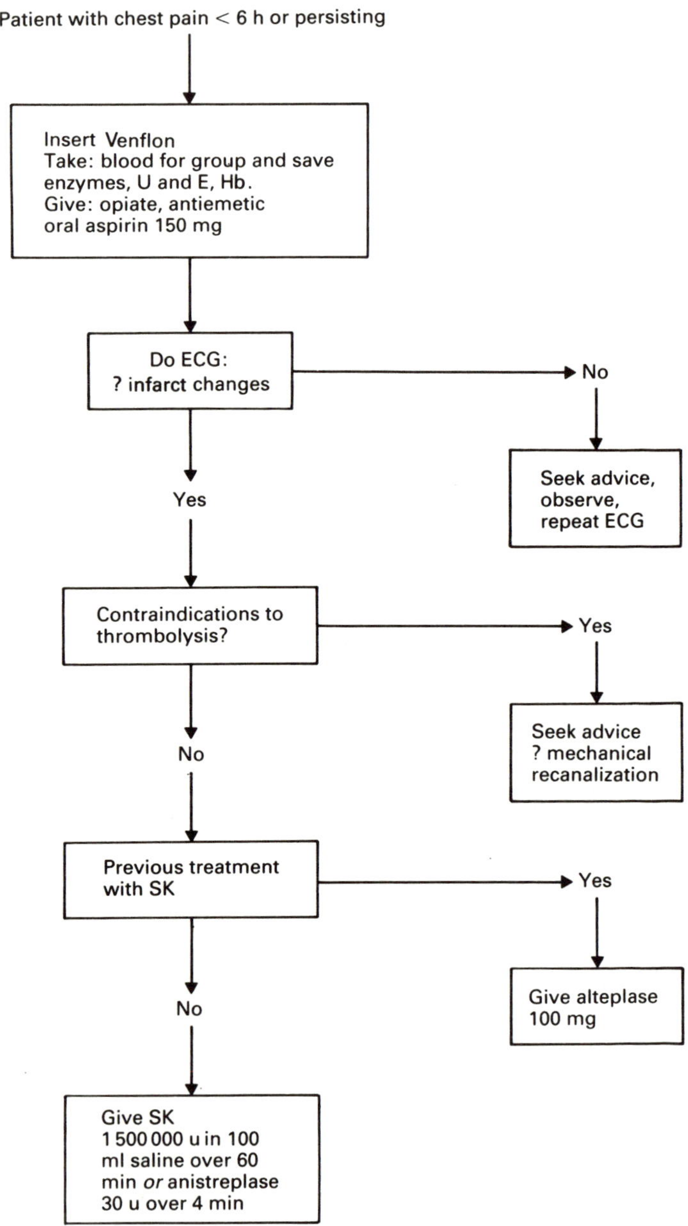

Fig. 12.1 Flow-chart for thrombolysis.

750000 vials) in 100 ml 0.9% NaCl is set up and scheduled to run over 1 hour. At 0900 Mr J.C. is transferred to the CCU. At 0920 there is a short run of accelerated idioventricular rhythm, and a repeat ECG shows a marked diminution of ST elevation. A repeat fibrinogen measurement at 1500 shows a fall from 4.5 g/litre on admission to 0.8 g/litre. At 0930 his blood pressure is 95 systolic, pulse 70/minute, he is warm and well perfused. A decision is made not to give intravenous betablockers. His subsequent CCU course is uneventful and he is transferred to a medical ward next day taking aspirin 150 mg/day and timolol 5 mg b.d. Plasma creatine kinase was 650 units/litre at 5 p.m., on the first day, and subsequently declined rapidly. The ECG evolved to show small Q waves in V2 and V3, with terminal T inversion. He was discharged home after 7 days.

At outpatient review a month later, he was well but had chest pain on climbing stairs. An exercise test was positive at stage 5 of the Bruce protocol. Subsequent angiography showed a stenosed left anterior descending coronary artery, and he underwent successful coronary angioplasty.

Example 2

Mrs G.M., aged 64, was admitted to a general medical ward at the request of her family practitioner at 1515. The previous day she had had an episode of chest pain at rest lasting 10 minutes, and this had re-occurred at 1000 that morning. Six months ago she had had an anterior myocardial infarct treated with intravenous streptokinase at another hospital. A month ago she developed angina of effort, and was awaiting cardiological assessment. Meanwhile she was taking propranolol 90 mg b.d.

On arrival in the ward she was undistressed, BP 130/92, pulse 65 and the rest of the examination was normal. ECG showed sinus rhythm and left bundle-branch block. Blood was taken for haemoglobin, white count, platelets, cardiac enzymes and electrolytes. A provisional diagnosis of unstable angina was made, propranolol was continued and nifedipine and aspirin added.

At 2200 she complained of chest pain which rapidly got worse, despite oral and then intravenous glyceryl trinitrate. She was vasoconstricted and the blood pressure fell to 105/72. The ECG still showed left bundle-branch block. At 2230 a decision was made to start thrombolytic therapy. Alteplase 100 mg was given as a 10 mg bolus, 50 mg over 1 hour and 20 mg after each of the next 2 hours. Heparin was given as a bolus of 5000 units, followed by 1000 m/hour. Morphine 10 mg and cyclizine 50 mg was also given. At 2330 pain had abated and she was sleeping quietly. The next morning a blood sample gave a thrombin/calcium coagulation time of 60 seconds compared to a control of 19 seconds, and the heparin dose was reduced to 800 units/hour. The initial set of cardiac enzyme levels were normal, but subsequently there was a small rise to a maximum creatine kinase activity of 400 units/litre.

The convalescence was uneventful and she was discharged 8 days after admission. Heparin was continued for 72 hours then stopped. She was sent home on propranolol, nifedipine and aspirin, with arrangements for elective coronary angiography in 3 weeks. This showed good left ventricular function with a patent but stenosed left anterior descending coronary artery, and severe stenosis on the right and circumflex coronaries. An exercise test was positive, and she eventually had coronary artery grafting.

Example 3

Mr D.L., aged 52, was transferred to a cardiology unit from a general hospital because of the unstable angina developing 7 days after cholecystectomy. Coronary arteriography at 1100 showed a stenosis of the left anterior descending coronary artery. The catheter was withdrawn and haemostasis secured. At 2100 he developed severe chest pain and features of anterior myocardial infarction. Thrombolysis was contraindicated because of: (a) recent abdominal surgery; and (b) the recent arterial puncture. Instead the patient was taken back to the catheter laboratory, where repeat catheterization showed total occlusion of the left anterior descending artery. He was given 150 mg aspirin to chew and 10 000 of heparin intravenously. An angioplasty guiding catheter was inserted and the blockage probed and crossed with a fine guidewire. Following this, 'ghost filling' of the distal left anterior descending artery could be seen on contrast injection. An angioplasty balloon was passed over the guidewire and the residual stenosis dilated. An arterial sheath was left in the femoral artery after withdrawal of the angioplasty catheter, guidewire and guiding catheter. Heparin was started at 1000 mg/hour 6 hours after the procedure, and continued until the following day. The sheath was removed 4 hours after stopping the heparin, and the subsequent course was uneventful.

Comment

Shows the use of an alternative therapy (acute angioplasty) where thrombolysis was contraindicated. A case could be made for leaving a femoral artery sheath *in situ* after diagnostic angiography in unstable angina.

13: Alternatives to Thrombolysis

Intravenous thrombolytic therapy is the treatment of choice for the vast majority of patients with acute myocardial infarction. In a few specific instances however other forms of treatment may be preferable for reasons of efficacy or safety. The three possible alternatives are:

1 Intracoronary administration of thrombolytics.
2 Mechanical recanalization and angioplasty.
3 Immediate coronary bypass surgery.

Intracoronary thrombolysis

In terms of efficacy in securing reperfusion, intracoronary thrombolytic therapy is equal to the best that can be attained using intravenous thrombolysis. Its disadvantages are the delay involved in taking the patient to the catheter room, the need for angiographic facilities, and the requirement for arterial cannulation. These disadvantages need not apply in the case of patients who sustain a coronary occlusion while already inpatients in a cardiology unit, but with the increasing availability of skilled operators, direct mechanical recanalization and angioplasty (as discussed below) may be an even more attractive option.

Original hopes that intracoronary thrombolytic therapy with non-fibrin-selective agents such as streptokinase would cause fewer haemorrhagic complications than intravenous therapy with larger doses of the same agents, remain unproven. Even with a relatively small dose of 250 000 units of streptokinase as commonly used for intracoronary thrombolysis, there is often a profound fall in plasma fibrinogen concentration. Data on the intracoronary use of fibrin selective agents are even more limited.

In our own experience, intracoronary infusion of 5–10 units of anistreplase caused little systemic fibrinogen depletion, and similar results have been reported for alteplase: the relative fibrin selectivity of agents tends to be greater with smaller doses. However patient numbers are too small for this to be reliably related to bleeding risk, and overall studies which have involved cardiac catheterization have tended to produce much higher rates of bleeding complications than those which have not.

One situation where intracoronary thrombolysis remains attractive, and is indeed the management of choice, is in the treatment of an acutely thrombosed aorto–coronary saphenous vein graft (see p. 98).

Mechanical perforation and angioplasty

Historically, mechanical perforation of a thrombotic coronary obstruction followed by angioplasty of the residual stenosis, was introduced as an adjunct to intracoronary thrombolytic therapy. Technical developments in angioplasty, and in particular the advent of steerable wire guided balloons, soon led to its independent use without a thrombolytic drug. O'Neill and colleagues found that immediate elective angioplasty was more effective than intravenous streptokinase in securing coronary patency in acute myocardial infarction, with a lower degree of residual coronary stenosis and better preservation of left ventricular function. The question as to why angioplasty *without* thrombolytic therapy appears to be effective and safe, whereas angioplasty as an immediate adjunct to thrombolysis seems to convey no advantage and may increase side-effects, has exercised a number of authors. There is some evidence that the risk of vascular intramural haemorrhage is increased if thrombolysis and angioplasty are combined; it is also possible that patients chosen for immediate angioplasty without thrombosis tend to be a 'good risk' group with a relatively short ischaemic period.

The most promising group of patients for direct mechanical recanalization are (as already discussed) those who actually develop coronary occlusion while inpatients in a cardiology unit. This group will contain a relatively high proportion of patients admitted with unstable angina, and perhaps also patients with reocclusion after successful initial thrombolytic therapy. Mechanical recanalization should also be considered in patients with a major contraindication to thrombolysis, such as early pregnancy, recent major surgery, or known peptic ulceration.

Mechanical recanalization is contraindicated when there is extensive intracoronary thrombus, which might be displaced distally or proximally. This applies especially to patients with thrombosed aorto–coronary vein grafts.

Case description

A 57-year-old man was admitted with unstable angina. A saphenous vein aortocoronary bypass operation had been performed a year earlier, with the left anterior descending as one of the grafted vessels. Angiography revealed patency of all the major vessels, but there appeared to be a tight proximal stenosis of the LAD graft. An attempt was made to angioplasty this site. Following balloon inflation, the patient complained of chest pain and developed anterior T wave changes on the ECG. Repeat angiography revealed that a considerable proportion of the 'stenosis' was in fact thrombus, and had been displaced distally into the LAD vessel. The patient was treated with intracoronary streptokinase, and angiography the next day showed clearing of the thrombus. Angioplasty was eventually performed to relieve the residual stenosis.

Mechanical recanalization may be impracticable if vascular access is prevented by severe peripheral atheroma.

The role of mechanical recanalization in patients with failed reperfusion after thrombolytic therapy is controversial. There is consistent evidence that patients who fail to reperfuse are at increased risk of death and of serious impairment of left ventricular function. However, as discussed elsewhere (p. 16), the ECSG trial provided no evidence of benefit from a policy of early elective angiography and intervention. Whether results would be improved by a more selective intervention policy based on non-invasive detection of continued occlusion, by better angioplasty techniques, or by using better anticoagulants such as antibodies to the platelet $GPII_b/III_a$ complex constitutes a series of questions which one day may be resolved by trials. Meanwhile, it would be appropriate to try mechanical re-canalization in anyone with continuing ischaemic pain and persistent coronary occlusion 90 minutes after the start of thrombolysis.

Surgical revascularization

Acute surgical revascularization in myocardial infarction has had a long and controversial history. Some groups have shown consistent enthusiasm for this approach, and have demonstrated good results, albeit in relatively few patients. Other have tried very hard to avoid any kind of surgery in the peri-infarct period.

Apart from the obvious and major logistic questions of surgical availability, the success of surgical revascularization hinges on: (a) the speed of revascularization; and (b) the ability of critically ischaemic myocardium to withstand the additional rigours of surgery, manifested as either 'warm ischaemia' or the use of cold cardioplegic solutions. Modification of surgical technique to improve results with ischaemic myocardium is under active investigation. Meanwhile, the major role for surgical revascularization appears to be in patients who develop sudden and irreversible coronary occlusion during attempted angioplasty—though even here, its benefit has not been unequivocally documented. In the author's experience of such cases, the results of surgery tend to be much better if there is at least some preservation of distal flow pre-operatively.

Further reading

O'Neill, W.W., Timmis, G.C., Bourdillon, P.D. *et al.* (1986). A prospective randomised clinical trial of intracoronary streptokinase versus coronary angioplasty for acute myocardial infarction. *New England Journal of Medicine*, **314**, 812–818.

14: Thrombolysis of Coronary Artery Grafts

A proportion of coronary artery vein grafts fail by thrombosis.

Early graft thrombosis

If a graft thromboses soon after surgery, there is usually still a residual blood supply to the myocardium through the stenosed but still patent native vessel, so the patient tends to present, not with myocardial infarction, but with a sudden recurrence of previous angina. These patients should be investigated as a matter of urgency, because if thrombolysis can be accomplished before the thrombus has organized, it may be possible to save the graft. Early graft thrombosis nearly always occurs in a graft which is stenosed, usually as a consequence of a technical problem at the time of surgery, and it may be possible to relieve the stenosis by angioplasty.

This is one of the few occasions where intracoronary thrombolysis may have an advantage: there is time to arrange angiography because myocardium is not immediately at risk, angiography will enable the state of the whole coronary tree and the other grafts to be assessed properly, and the catheter can be used to direct a thrombolytic drug into the middle of the thrombus, which is usually much larger than the thrombi occurring in native coronary vessels.

CASE DESCRIPTION

A 70-year-old man had had saphenous vein bypass grafts to the left anterior descending and right coronary arteries 10 weeks previously. He presented with a sudden recurrence of his angina, and his ECG showed new T wave inversion in the inferior leads. Coronary arteriography showed a patent right coronary artery with a tight proximal stenosis, and a graft to this vessel which was occluded by thrombus 3 cm from its origin. The 7 FG right Judkins catheter used to enter the graft was left *in situ* and a 2.5 FG infusion catheter advanced into the centre of the thrombus. Streptokinase was infused at approximately 2000 units/minute through the infusion catheter. The patient was returned to the coronary care unit with the catheter *in situ* and the progress of graft clearance followed cautiously by injecting small quantities of contrast medium through the catheter. After 2 hours the graft was fully patent, but angiography showed a tight stenosis at its lower end which was treated with angioplasty. The stenosis in the proximal right coronary artery was also dilated.

Late graft thrombosis

Late thrombosis of a coronary graft is more likely to lead to infarction, because the native vessel may no longer be patent. Patients may also of course have infarction because disease has progressed in a native vessel. A patient who suffers acute infarction late after coronary bypass grafting should be given intravenous thrombolytic therapy in the usual way (see Chapters 4–6) and should then have follow-up angiography to evaluate the situation. It may sometimes be possible to clear thrombus from an old graft, but the suitability of 'old grafts' for angioplasty needs to be assessed carefully: some have a very friable intima which fragments during angioplasty and can lead to distal embolic complications.

Summary

- Patients with an early recurrence of angina after coronary grafting should have urgent angiography.
- Graft thrombus can be cleared by thrombolytic therapy: intracoronary administration may be the best approach.
- Early graft thrombosis usually indicates graft stenosis, which many need angioplasty.
- Patients presenting with infarction should have intravenous thrombolysis first, then proceed to angiography.

15: Thrombolysis for other Conditions

Although the primary aim of this book is to describe thrombolysis for acute myocardial infarction, it would be incomplete to omit entirely a discussion of other potential uses of thrombolytic therapy. For the majority of these, although there is often convincing anecdotal evidence of efficacy, the sheer weight of evidence and experience which exists for thrombolysis in myocardial infarction is lacking. It is even more important, therefore, to consider each case on its merits and to balance very carefully the potential benefits against the hazards.

Pulmonary embolism

There have been a large number of trials of thrombolytic therapy in pulmonary embolism, but the total number of patients has been relatively small. There is evidence that thrombolytic therapy improves the rate of improvement of the pulmonary angiographic score, and that it accelerates the return to normal of cardiac output and pulmonary artery pressure, but no formal demonstration that it improves survival. This is however, to some extent, an artefact of trial design, in that in a number of studies clinical deterioration was an indication to break randomization and allocate the patient to thrombolytic therapy. There is a consensus that patients with a definite diagnosis of massive pulmonary embolism who have a raised jugular venous pressure, hypotension (systolic < 100 mmHg) and hypoxaemia (arterial $Po_2 < 10$ KPa on oxygen) should be considered for thrombolysis. The contraindications are the general ones to thrombolytic therapy listed in Chapter 4. All the major thrombolytic agents have been shown to be effective in pulmonary embolism, but only streptokinase and urokinase are presently licensed for this indication in the UK. The currently recommended dose schedules are listed in Table 15.1. Although it has been traditional to give prolonged infusions of thrombolytic agents, recent work suggests that short-term or bolus infusions may give similar efficacy with fewer bleeding complications.

Ideally, the diagnosis should be confirmed by angiography before starting thrombolysis, but this is not an excuse for delay in treating a deteriorating patient. Bedside echocardiography will often provide strong evidence for pulmonary embolism in the form of a dilated right ventricle and right ventricular outflow tract (sometimes with visible thrombus) and a small, underfilled and vigorously contracting left ventricle. Catheterization and angiography does have the advantage that the passage of a catheter into the pulmonary artery may help to break up thrombus, and there have been reports that this can be done more effectively with a balloon catheter of the type used for pulmonary valvuloplasty. The best site for introducing a catheter is via an antecubital vein (see Chapter 16), and it should be left *in situ* in the pulmonary artery during thrombolysis to monitor pulmonary artery pressure, and to permit follow-up angiography 12 hours after starting treatment.

Table 15.1 Dose regimes in pulmonary embolism.

Streptokinase
250 000 u over 30 min followed by 100 000 u/h for 24 h (ref. *Journal of the American Medical Association*, (1974) **229**, 1606–1613.)

Urokinase
(a) 4400 u/kg over 30 min followed by 4400 u/kg/h over 12–24 h (ref. *Circulation* (1973) **47**, (2), 1–108) *OR* (b) single bolus of 20 000 u/kg. (ref. *Circulation* (1984) **70**, 861–866)

Alteplase
50 mg over 2 h followed by 10 mg/h for 4 h (ref. *Lancet* (1986) **ii**, 886–889)

Anistreplase
30 u i.v. over 4 min (no published data on use in pulmonary embolism)

These dose schedules have been described in the literature, but the agents are not necessarily licensed for use in pulmonary embolism.

Follow-up anticoagulation with intravenous heparin has been usual after thrombolysis for pulmonary embolism. The optimal time for starting heparin is best decided in consultation with a blood coagulation laboratory. Warfarin is usually started after 5–7 days and heparin discontinued once the prothrombin time ratio is stable.

Deep vein thrombosis

The conventional treatment of deep venous thrombosis is with intravenous heparin. Mortality from this condition is low, but there is a risk that extensive iliofemoral thrombosis will be followed by chronic venous insufficiency ('post-phlebitic leg' syndrome). There is some evidence that thrombolytic therapy will accelerate clearance of the thrombus and reduce the incidence of chronic venous insufficiency, but at the cost of an increased risk of haemorrhage. Streptokinase has been the most widely used agent, though alteplase is also effective.

Peripheral arterial thrombosis

Early studies in the use of streptokinase to relieve peripheral arterial thrombosis achieved moderate success at the cost of a high morbidity from bleeding. The development of the Fogarty balloon embolectomy/thrombectomy catheter led for a while to a virtual abandonment of arterial thrombolysis, but recently it is experiencing something of a resurgence in popularity, particularly for limb salvage after thrombosis of the femoral artery and femoro-popliteal grafts. A factor in this has been the development, initially by Dotter and subsequently by McNamara and colleagues, of a technique of infusing a thrombolytic agent directly into the thrombus through a fine catheter (Fig. 15.1, and see Chapter 13). The original literature should be consulted for technical details. Angioplasty may subsequently be performed to relieve residual stenoses.

Thrombosed artificial heart valves

Mechanical heart valve prostheses are prone to undergo thrombosis unless the patient is anticoagulated. Frequently the

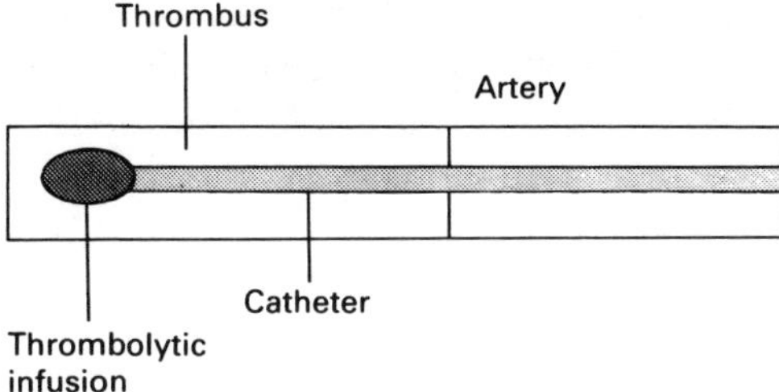

Fig. 15.1 Dotter–McNamara technique for direct infusion of thrombolytics into intra-arterial thrombus.

thrombosis is only detected when the valve becomes stuck and the patient undergoes a catastrophic decline in cardiac output. In these circumstances emergency surgery is the only realistic option. In a few cases however, thrombosis can be detected at an earlier stage because of abnormal muffling of the valve clicks and echocardiographic evidence of impaired function. Thrombolytic therapy may be effective in these circumstances.

Stroke

The ability of a small thrombus to cause major functional impairment is demonstrated even more spectacularly in the brain than in the heart. Thrombolytic therapy for stroke has however to cope with two major drawbacks — the difficulty of distinguishing clinically between thrombosis/embolism and haemorrhage, and the tendency for cerebral haemorrhage to complicate cerebral infarction. The first problem is capable of being overcome with the more widespread use of computerized tomographic scanning — this will not detect early infarction, but will detect early haemorrhage with a high degree of accuracy. The second problem is increasingly recognized to be a function of the time between occlusion of the vessel and reperfusion: occlusion times of more than 2 hours are more likely to be followed by haemorrhage on reperfusion. There have been fascinating animal studies and a limited number of clinical case reports on thrombolytic therapy in stroke, and this is likely to be a major field for future development.

Unstable angina

Unstable angina is defined as anginal type chest pain coming on at rest or on minimal physical activity, particularly when there is a progressive reduction over a short period of time in the amount of activity which induces the symptoms. Electrocardiogram may show ST segment elevation or depression or alteration in T wave shape during the episodes of pain but there are no permanent electrocardiographic changes and there is no elevation of the cardiac enzymes.

Unstable angina is frequently due to the rupture of an atherosclerotic plaque with the associate formation of a variable amount of thrombus which narrows the coronary lumen but does not permanently occlude it. Because this is exactly the same process as that which leads to occlusive coronary thrombosis, and ultimately myocardial infarction, there will be a stage at which it is impossible to distinguish clinically between unstable angina and impending myocardial infarction. It is only as the time course of the clinical and electrocardiographic changes becomes apparent that the diagnosis can be made. Patients admitted to a hospital or CCU with a diagnosis of unstable angina constitute a selected population in which the progression of coronary occlusion is relatively slow. Of these patients, 15–20% may progress to myocardial infarction while in the remainder the situation stabilizes, presumably as a result of organization of the disrupted atheromatous plaque and the spontaneous disillusion or organization of the thrombus.

Patients with unstable angina are more likely to progress to myocardial infarction. This may occur if there are major or prolonged ECG T wave changes during pain, if the ECG fails to return to normal between attacks of pain, if the attacks of pain are frequent and persistent despite medical therapy, and if continuous ECG monitoring shows frequent episodes of ST segment elevation or depression even in the absence of pain. The risk of infarction is reduced by the use of the aspirin, heparin or a combination of the two, and outcome is also improved by beta-blockade. Oral or intravenous nitrates or nifedipine help to provide symptomatic relief but evidence they improve prognosis is lacking. Most cardiac centres proceed to coronary arteriography with a view to either angioplasty or coronary artery grafting if symptoms of unstable angina persist in spite of medical therapy.

The role of thrombolytic therapy in unstable angina is unproven. On one hand the mechanistic analogy with myocardial infarction and the unequivocal demonstration of intracoronary thrombus by either angiography or angioscopy make it logical, on the other hand it seems likely that in patients with unstable angina who present to hospital, the pathophysiological balance is already tilted against the extensive propagation of thrombus. Clinical trials have so far been small scale, and have reflected this uncertainty. In a study by Gold and colleagues, thrombolytic therapy was helpful in patients where there was angiographic evidence of thrombus, but not in a similar proportion of patients who had no clear-cut evidence of it. This distinction is not particularly helpful clinically. A large scale clinical trial in the USA (TIMI-3) is attempting to evaluate the role of thrombolytic therapy in unstable angina on a formal basis. The use of thrombolytic agents as an adjutant to angioplasty in unstable angina is again logical, but is at present based solely on anecdotal evidence.

Further reading

Pulmonary embolism

Meyer, G., Sors, H., Charbonnier, B., Brochier, M.L. & Stern, M. (1989) Thrombolysis in acute pulmonary embolism. In Julian, D., Kubler, W., Norris, R.M. *et al. Thrombolysis in Cardiovascular Disease*. Marcel Dekker, New York, pp. 337–360.

Miller, G.A.H., Sutton, G.C., Kerr, I.H., Gibson, R.V. & Honey, M. (1971) Comparison of streptokinase and urokinase in the treatment of isolated acute massive pulmonary embolism. *British Medical Journal*, **ii**, 681–684.

Tibbutt, D.A., Davis, J.A., Anderson, J.A. *et al.* (1974) Comparison by controlled clinical trial of streptokinase and heparin in treatment of life threatening pulmonary embolism. *British Medical Journal*, **i**, 343–347.

Deep vein thrombosis

Goldhaber, S.Z., Buring, J.E., Lipnick, R.J. & Hennekens, C.H. (1984) Pooled analyses of randomised trials of streptokinase and heparin in phlebographically documented acute deep venous thrombosis. *American Journal of Medicine*, **76**, 393–397.

Peripheral arterial thrombosis

Graor, R.A., Risius, B., Young, J.R. *et al.* (1984) Low dose streptokinase for selective thrombolysis: systemic effects and complications. *Radiology*, **152**, 35–40.

McNamara, T.O. & Bomberger, R.A. (1986) Factors affecting initial and six month patency following high dose intraarterial urokinase thrombolysis. *American Journal of Surgery*, **152**, 709–712.

Verstraete, M., Hess, H., Mahler, F. *et al.* (1988) Femoropopliteal artery thrombolysis with intra-arterial infusion of recombinant tissue type plasminogen activator: report of a pilot trial. *European Journal of Vascular Surgery*, **2**, 155–159.

Thrombosed artificial heart valves

Ledain, L.D., Ohayon, J.P., Colle, J.P., Lorient Roudaut, F.M., Roudaut, R.M. & Besse, P.M. (1986) Acute thrombotic obstruction with disc valve prostheses: diagnostic considerations and thrombolytic treatment. *Journal of the American College of Cardiology*, **7**, 743–751.

Unstable angina

Gold, H.K. (1989) Thrombolysis in patients with unstable angina. In Julian, D., Kubler, W., Norris, R.M., Swan, H.J.C., Collen, D. & Verstraete, M. (eds) *Thrombolysis in Cardiovascular Disease*. Marcel Dekker, New York, pp. 325–336.

16: Vascular Procedures in Patients undergoing Thrombolytic Therapy

Recent puncture of an artery or other non-compressible major vessel has been described earlier as a contraindication to thrombolysis. However it is quite often necessary, in patients with myocardial infarction, to gain vascular access to insert a pacing electrode, Swan–Ganz catheter, or even to perform coronary arteriography. This chapter describes how these procedures can be performed safely. The techniques are summarized in Table 16.1.

Venepuncture

'In and out' venepuncture, even with a small needle, will cause bleeding. It is better to put an in-dwelling cannula ('Venflon' or similar) of reasonable size, e.g. 16 gauge, into an accessible arm vein and to use this both for drug administration and blood sampling. The cannula should be flushed well with saline after

Table 16.1 Vascular procedures in patients undergoing thrombolysis.

Venepuncture
Insert single in-dwelling cannula ('Venflon' or similar), anchor firmly with tape, flush twice daily with saline

Arterial puncture (for blood gas or pressure monitoring)
Avoid if possible. If essential use in-dwelling cannula in radial or femoral artery, remove when thrombolytic activity has ceased

Central venous access (pacing, Swan–Ganz catheter)
Use antecubital (basilic) vein if possible. Alternatives femoral or jugular. Avoid subclavian

Cardiac catheterization coronary arteriography
Femoral approach with in-dwelling sheath(s) or brachial approach with direct suture

use, and not allowed to remain in for longer than 48 hours. The systemic thrombolytic effect is usually over in 6–12 hours.

Arterial puncture

Avoid this if possible in the first 6–12 hours after thrombolysis. If essential, an in-dwelling 18 or 20 gauge radial artery cannula (in the non-dominant arm) is preferable, and it should be removed when haemostasis is stable.

Pacing electrodes and Swan–Ganz catheters

These can safely be inserted via an antecubital vein, using either a percutaneous technique or a small cut-down. Do not use the cephalic vein (lateral aspect of the antecubital fossa) as the catheter or electrode will not negotiate the kink as this joins the subclavian. Do not use direct subclavian puncture, as you cannot control bleeding either from the vein or from an inadvertently punctured artery. The internal jugular vein is a better approach, but only for the skilled and experienced operator, for example a cardiac anaesthetist. The safest alternative, if the antecubital route is impracticable, is to use the femoral vein. This does present problems of catheter stability and ease of nursing, but they can usually be overcome for a short period, and once the period of thrombolytic activity is over the catheter or pacing wire can be resited.

Cardiac catheterization

There are two equally satisfactory approaches to the problem of arterial catheterization during active thrombolytic therapy. The first is to use a brachial artery approach and to suture the artery under direct vision, the second is to use an arterial sheath inserted by the Seldinger technique and left *in situ* until thrombolytic activity has declined. If using a percutaneous approach, the aim should be to make a clean puncture of the anterior wall (only) of the femoral artery at a point where the puncture site can readily be compressed against the superior pubic ramus. An arterial sheath can be left *in situ* for up to 48 hours provided the patient is kept anticoagulated. To prevent accidental dislodgement, the sheath should be sutured to the skin. In obese patients a thin-walled sheath may buckle and it may be impossible to reinsert a catheter—the use of force may damage the wall of the sheath and cause bleeding. If repeat angiography is likely to be needed, it is wise to reinforce the sheath (and reduce the risk of intrasheath thrombus) by inserting an obturator.

Appendix: Ready Reference Pages

Table A1 Consensus criteria for initiating thrombolytic therapy in suspected infarction. (Based on ASSET and ISIS-2 criteria (1989).)

1 Strong clinical suspicion of myocardial infarction based on type, severity and duration of chest pain
2 At least some ECG evidence of myocardial ischaemia or infarction
3 Absence of major contraindications

Table A2 Current contraindications to thrombolysis in acute myocardial infarction.

Absolute
Active internal bleeding
Subarachnoid haemorrhage or intracerebral haemorrhage within 2 months

Relative major
Major surgery, obstetrical delivery, organ biopsy or puncture of non-compressible vessels within 10 days
Recent serious gastrointestinal bleeding
Recent serious trauma, including any head injury
Cerebral infarct within 48 h
Prolonged or traumatic cardiopulmonary resuscitation

Relative minor
Recent minor trauma
Pregnancy
Diabetic hemorrhagic and proliferative retinopathy
Age over 75 years

Table A3 Reversing thrombolysis.

1 Stop infusion of thrombolytic drug and/or heparin
2 Consult with blood coagulation laboratory if possible. Take samples for measurement of fibrinogen, euglobulin lysis time, reptilase time. Cross match blood
3 Give tranexamic acid 10 mg/kg i.v.
4 Give aprotinin (Trasylol, Bayer) 500 000 u over 10 min, then 200 000 u over 4 h
5 If fibrinogen < 1 g/l, consider giving fresh frozen plasma or fibrinogen concentrate

Table A4 Treatment of anaphylaxis.

1 Discontinue drug infusion
2 Hydrocortisone 100 mg plus chlorpheniramine 10 mg i.v.
3 Adrenaline 1/1000 (1 mg/ml) 0.5 ml (0.5 mg) subcutaneously, repeated if necessary
4 Adrenaline infusion 4 μg/ml (2 ml of 1/1000 adrenaline in 500 ml saline) titrated against response
5 Intubate and ventilate if necessary

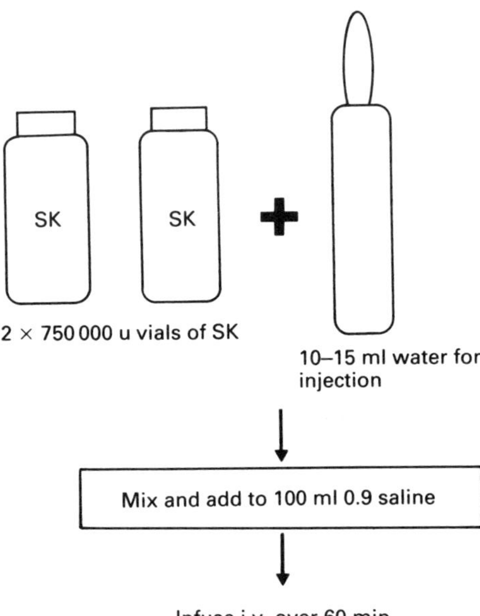

Fig. A1 Administration of streptokinase in acute myocardial infarction. Note that an alternative is to make up streptokinase as two injections of 750 000 u in 10 ml, each given over 5–10 min with a gap of 20 min.

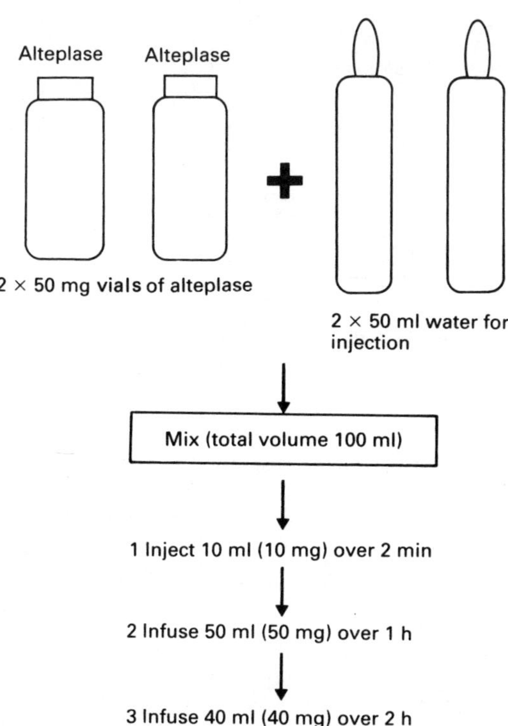

Fig. A2 Administration of alteplase in acute myocardial infarction. Note that if the patient weighs less than 67 kg, adjust dose to 1.5 mg/kg.

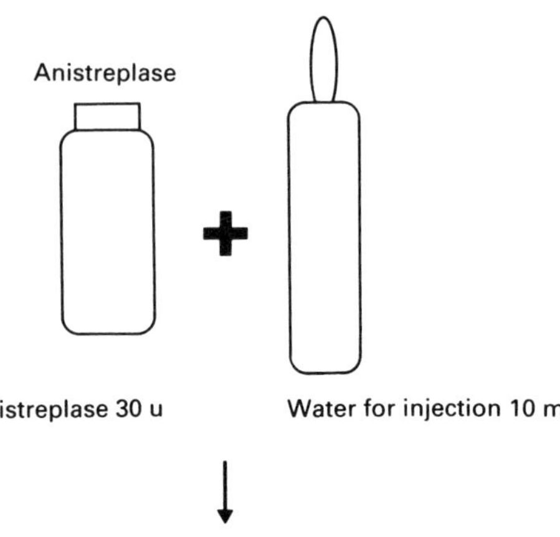

Fig. A3 Administration of anistreplase in acute myocardial infarction.

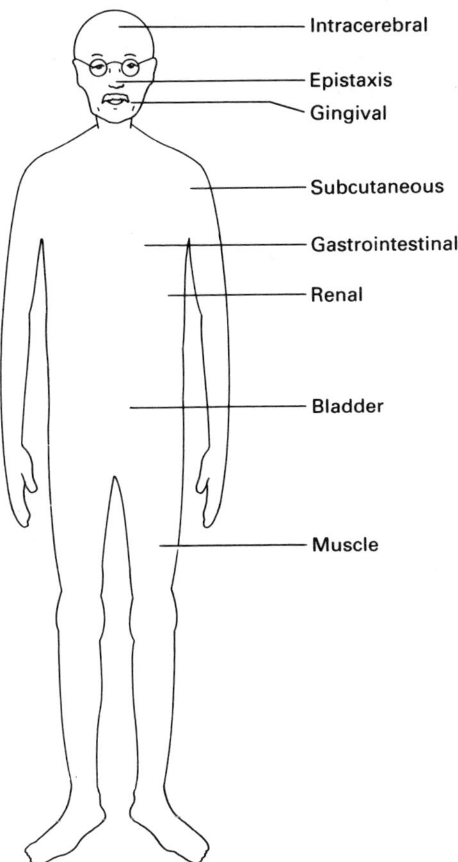

Fig. A4 Principal sites of spontaneous bleeding during thrombolysis.

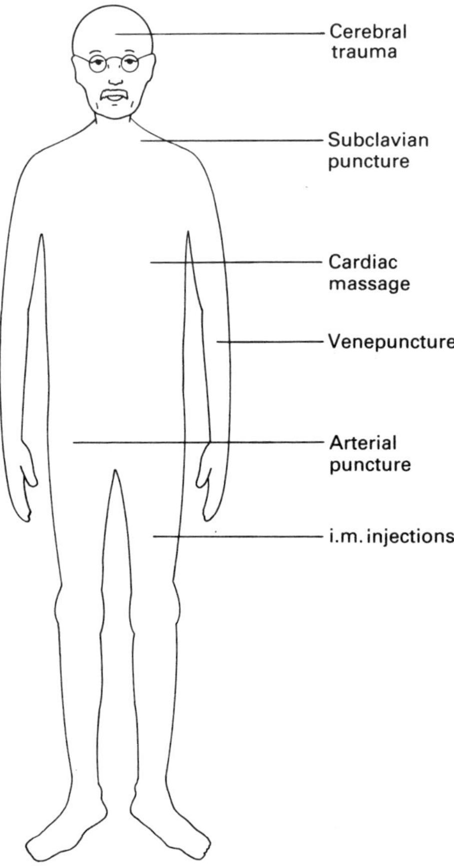

Fig. A5 Principal sites of iatrogenic haemorrhage during thrombolysis.

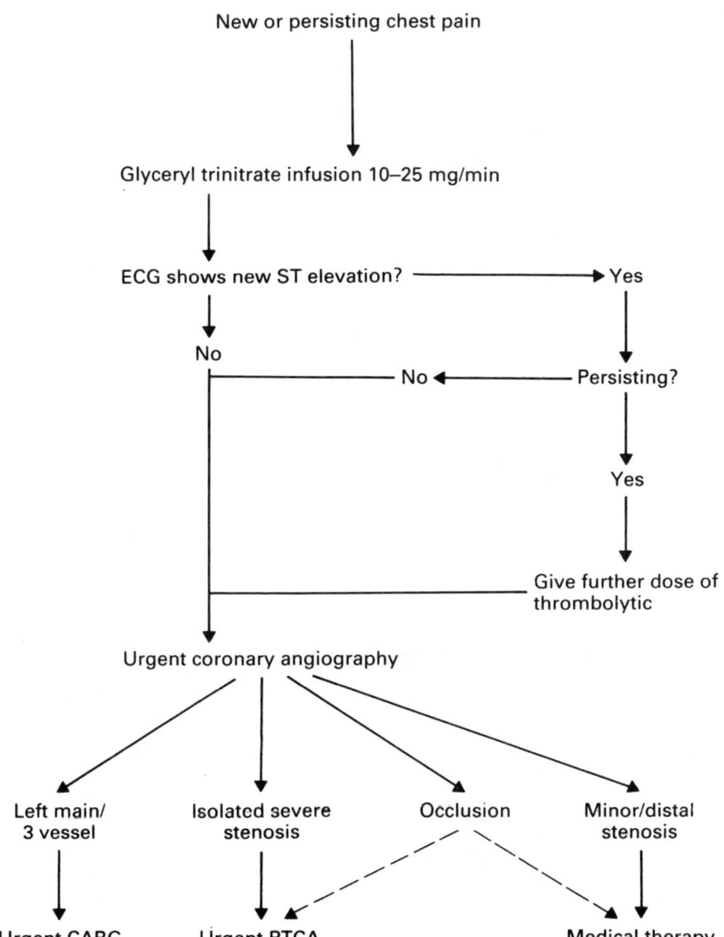

Fig. A6 Management of recurrent ischaemia after thrombolysis.

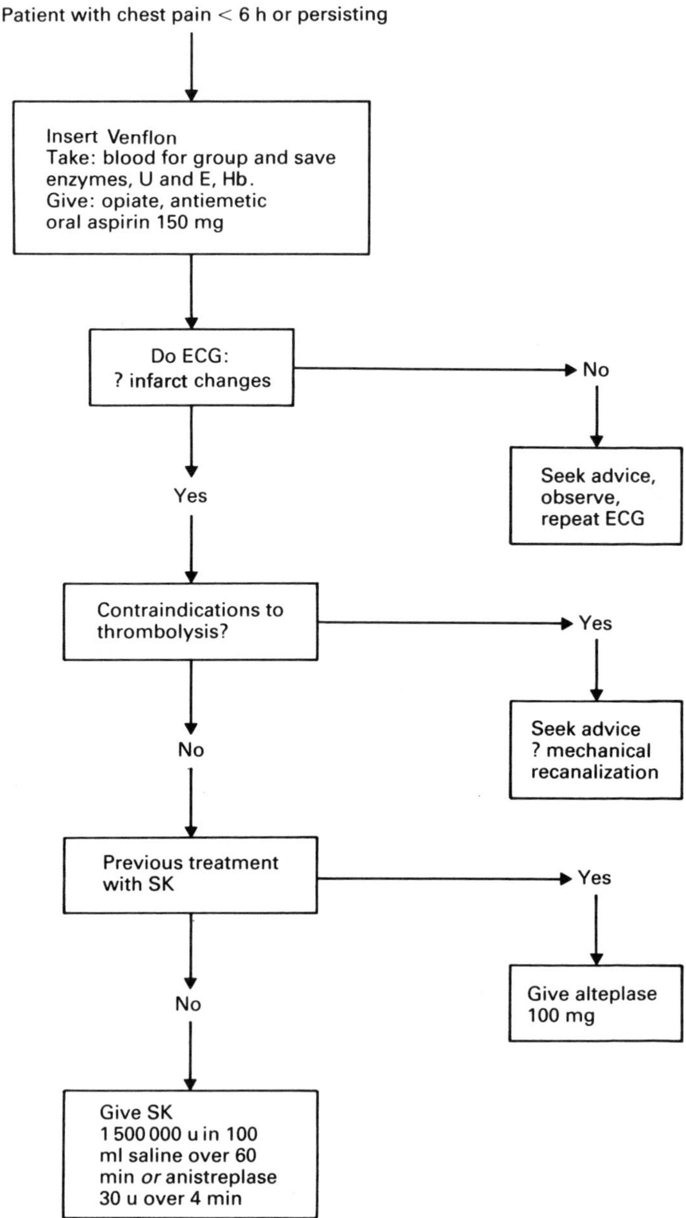

Fig. A7 Flow-chart for thrombolysis.

Index

Page numbers in *italics* indicate figures, and in **bold** indicate tables.